Thinking Good, Feeling Better

Thinking Good, Feeling Better

A Cognitive Behavioural Therapy Workbook for Adolescents and Young Adults

Paul Stallard

WILEY

Registered Offices
John Wiley & Sons, Inc., 111 River Street, Hoboken, NJ 07030, USA
John Wiley & Sons Ltd, The Atrium, Southern Gate, Chichester, West Sussex, PO19 8SQ, UK

Editorial Office
The Atrium, Southern Gate, Chichester, West Sussex, PO19 8SQ, UK

For details of our global editorial offices, customer services, and more information about Wiley products visit us at www.wiley.com.

Wiley also publishes its books in a variety of electronic formats and by print-on-demand. Some content that appears in standard print versions of this book may not be available in other formats.

Library of Congress Cataloging-in-Publication Data
Names: Stallard, Paul, 1955- author.
Title: Thinking good, feeling better : a cognitive behavioural therapy
    workbook for adolescents and young adults / Paul Stallard, Professor of
    Child and Family Mental Health, University of Bath, UK and Head of
    Psychological, Therapies (CAMHS), Oxford Health NHS Foundation Trust, UK.
Description: Hoboken, NJ : John Wiley & Sons, 2019. | Includes
    bibliographical references and index. |
Identifiers: LCCN 2018023895 (print) | LCCN 2018035282 (ebook) | ISBN
    9781119396284 (Adobe PDF) | ISBN 9781119397281 (ePub) | ISBN 9781119396291 (pbk.)
Subjects: LCSH: Behavior therapy for children. | Cognitive therapy for
    children. | Behavior therapy for teenagers. | Cognitive therapy for teenagers.
Classification: LCC RJ505.B4 (ebook) | LCC RJ505.B4 S72 2019 (print) | DDC
    618.92/89142–dc23
LC record available at https://lccn.loc.gov/2018023895

Cover Design: Wiley

Set in 10/13pt Legacy Sans by Thomson Digital, Noida, India
Printed and bound in Singapore by Markono Print Media Pte Ltd

Contents

About the author

Paul Stallard is Professor of Child and Family Mental Health at the University of Bath and Head of Psychological Therapies (CAMHS) for Oxford Health NHS Foundation Trust. He has worked with children and young people for over 30 years since qualifying as a clinical psychologist in Birmingham in 1980.

Clinically, Paul continues to work within a specialist child mental health team where he leads a Cognitive Behaviour Therapy (CBT) clinic for children and young people with a range of emotional disorders including anxiety, depression, obsessive compulsive disorder (OCD), and post-traumatic stress disorder (PTSD).

He is an international expert in the development and use of CBT with children and young people and has provided training in many countries. He is the author of the widely used *Think Good Feel Good: A Cognitive Behaviour Therapy Workbook for Children and Young People* and Editor of the book series *Cognitive Behaviour Therapy with Children, Adolescents and Families*.

He is an active researcher and has published widely in high-impact peer-reviewed journals. Recent research projects have included large school-based CBT programmes for depression and anxiety and the use of eHealth with children and young people.

Acknowledgement

There are many people who have directly and indirectly contributed to the development of this book.

First, I would like to thank my family, Rosie, Luke, and Amy for their encouragement and enthusiasm. Despite many long hours working, writing, and travelling, their support for this project has been unwavering.

Second, I have had the good fortune to work with many amazing colleagues during my career. A number of our clinical discussions have informed the ideas in this book. Of my colleagues, I would particularly like to thank Kate and Lucy who I have had the privilege to work with in our CBT clinic for over a decade. Their patience, creativity, and thoughtfulness have helped me to develop and test the ideas contained in this book.

Third, I would like to thank the children and young people I have had the honour to meet. Their determination to overcome their challenges continues to inspire and motivate me to find ways in which effective psychological interventions can be made more available.

Finally, I would like to thank those who read this book. I hope that these materials will help you to help a young person make a real difference to their life.

Online resources

All the text and workbook resources in this book are **available free, in colour, to purchasers** of the print version. To find out how to access and download these flexible aids to working with your clients visit the website

www.wiley.com/go/thinkinggood

The online facility provides an opportunity to download and print relevant sections of the workbook that can then be used in clinical sessions with young people. The materials can be used to structure or supplement clinical sessions or can be completed by the young person at home.

The online materials can be used flexibly, and can be accessed and used as often as required.

CHAPTER ONE

Cognitive behaviour therapy: theoretical origins, rationale, and techniques

Cognitive behaviour therapy (CBT) is a generic term used to describe a family of psychotherapeutic interventions that focus upon the relationship between cognitive, emotional, and behavioural processes. The overall aim of CBT is to facilitate an awareness of the important role of cognitions on emotions and behaviours (Hofmann, Sawyer, and Fang 2010). CBT therefore embraces the core elements of both cognitive and behavioural theories and has been defined by Kendall and Hollon (1979) as seeking to

> preserve the efficacy of behavioural techniques but within a less doctrinaire context that takes account of the child's cognitive interpretations and attributions about events.

> Cognitive Behaviour Therapy focuses upon the relationship between what we think (cognitions), how we feel (emotions), and what we do (behaviour).

The first randomised controlled trials demonstrating the effectiveness of CBT for children and adolescents emerged in the early 1900s (Lewinsohn et al. 1990; Kendall 1994). Numerous trials have since been reported resulting in CBT becoming established as the most extensively researched of all the child psychotherapies (Graham 2005). Reviews have found CBT to be an effective intervention for children and adolescents with a range of problems including anxiety (James et al. 2013; Reynolds et al. 2012; Fonagy et al. 2014), depression (Chorpita et al. 2011; Zhou et al. 2015; Thapar et al. 2012), post-traumatic stress disorder (Cary and McMillen 2012; Gillies et al. 2013), chronic pain (Palermo et al. 2010; Fisher et al. 2014), and obsessive compulsive disorder (Franklin et al. 2015). The substantial body of knowledge demonstrating effectiveness has resulted in CBT being recommended by expert groups such as the UK National Institute for Health and Clinical Excellence and the American Academy of Child and Adolescent Psychiatry for the treatment of young people with emotional disorders including depression, obsessive compulsive disorders, post-traumatic stress disorder, and anxiety. This growing evidence base has also prompted the development of a national training programme in the United Kingdom in CBT, Improving Access to Psychological Therapies (IAPT), which has now been extended to children and young people (Shafran et al. 2014).

> CBT is an empirically supported psychological intervention.

Thinking Good, Feeling Better: A Cognitive Behavioural Therapy Workbook for Adolescents and Young Adults, First Edition.
Paul Stallard.
© 2019 John Wiley & Sons Ltd. Published 2019 by John Wiley & Sons Ltd.
Companion website: www.wiley.com/go/thinkinggood

▶ The foundations of CBT

CBT describes a family of interventions that have evolved over time through three main phases or waves. The first wave was behaviour therapy which focused directly on the relationship between behaviour and emotions. Through the use of learning theory, new behaviours could be learned to replace those that are unhelpful. The second wave, cognitive therapy, built upon behavioural therapy by focusing on the subjective meanings and interpretations that are made about the events that occur. Directly challenging and testing the content of the biases that underpin these cognitions results in alternative, more helpful, balanced, and functional ways of thinking. Third wave CBT focuses on changing the nature of our relationship with our thoughts and emotions rather than actively attempting to change them. Thoughts and feelings are observed as inevitable mental and cognitive process rather than evidence of reality. Third wave models include Acceptance and Commitment Therapy (ACT), Compassion Focused Therapy (CFT), Dialectical Behaviour Therapy (DBT), and Mindfulness-based Cognitive Behaviour Therapy (MCBT).

▶ First wave: behaviour therapy

One of the earliest influences on the development of CBT was that of Pavlov (1927) and classical conditioning. Pavlov highlighted how, with repeated pairings, naturally occurring responses (e.g. salivation) could become associated (i.e. conditioned) with specific stimuli (e.g. the sound of a bell). The work demonstrated that emotional responses, such as fear, could become conditioned with specific events and situations such as snakes or crowded places.

> Emotional responses are associated with specific events.

Classical conditioning was extended to human behaviour and clinical problems by Wolpe (1958) who developed the procedure of systematic desensitisation. By pairing fear-inducing stimuli (e.g. watching a snake) with a second stimulus that produces an antagonistic response (i.e. relaxation) the fear response can be reciprocally inhibited. The procedure is now widely used in clinical practice and involves graded exposure, both in vivo and in imagination, to a hierarchy of feared situations whilst remaining relaxed.

> Emotional responses can be changed.

The second major behavioural influence was the work of Skinner (1974) who highlighted the significant role of environmental influences upon behaviour. This became known as operant conditioning and focused upon the relationship between antecedents (setting conditions), consequences (reinforcement), and behaviour. In essence, if a particular behaviour increased in occurrence because it is followed by positive consequences, or is not followed by negative consequences, then the behaviour has been reinforced. Behaviour could therefore be changed by altering the consequences or the conditions that evoked them.

> Altering antecedents and consequences can change behaviour.

Recognition of the mediating role of cognitive processes was noted by Bandura (1977) and the development of social learning theory. The role of the environment was recognised, but behaviour therapy was extended to highlight the importance of the cognitions that intervene between stimuli and response. The theory demonstrated that learning could occur through watching someone else and proposed a model of self-control based upon self-observation, self-evaluation, and self-reinforcement.

▶ Second wave: cognitive therapy

Behaviour therapy proved very effective, although it was criticised for failing to pay sufficient attention to the meanings and interpretations that are made about the events that occur. This stimulated interest in the development of cognitive therapy with a direct focus on the way individual's process and interpret events and the effect of these on emotions and behaviour.

This phase was heavily influenced by the pioneering work of Ellis (1962) and Beck (1963, 1964). Ellis (1962) developed Rational Emotive Therapy which was based upon the central relationship between cognitions and emotions. The model proposed that emotion and behaviour arise from the way events are construed rather than by the event per se. Thus activating events (A), are assessed against beliefs (B) that result in emotional consequences (C). Beliefs can be either rational or irrational with negative emotional states tending to arise from, and be maintained by, irrational beliefs.

Cognitions and emotions are linked.

The role of maladaptive and distorted cognitions in the development and maintenance of depression was developed through the work of Beck culminating in the publication of *Cognitive Therapy for Depression* (Beck 1976; Beck et al. 1979). The model proposes that emotional problems arise through biased cognitive processing in which events are distorted in negative and unhelpful ways. Underlying these biased ways of thinking are core beliefs or schemas. These are global, fixed, and rigid ways of thinking that are assumed to develop during childhood. Beliefs are activated by events reminiscent of those that produced them, and once activated, attention, memory, and interpretation processing biases filter and select information to support them. Attention biases result in attention being focused upon information that confirms the belief, whilst neutral or contradictory information is overlooked. Memory biases result in the recall of information that is consistent with the belief, whilst interpretation biases serve to minimise any inconsistent information.

Biased and distorted cognitions generate unpleasant emotions.

Once activated, fixed beliefs produce a range of automatic thoughts, the most accessible level of cognitions. Automatic thoughts or 'self-talk' represent the involuntary stream of thoughts that race through our heads providing a continuous commentary about the events that occur. These automatic thoughts tend to be about the self, the world, and the future, commonly referred to as the cognitive triad.

Beliefs are functionally related to automatic thoughts, resulting in biased and distorted beliefs producing negative automatic thoughts. Negative automatic thoughts are very self-critical and generate unpleasant emotional states, e.g. anxiety, anger, unhappiness, and unhelpful behaviours such as social withdrawal or avoidance.

The unpleasant feelings and unhelpful behaviours associated with these dysfunctional cognitions and processing biases serve to reinforce and maintain the original beliefs as the individual becomes trapped in a self-perpetuating negative cycle. The relationship between cognitive processes and other emotional states and psychological problems has been well documented (Beck 2005).

Interventions aim to identify and challenge the specific content of biased cognitions and processes in order to develop more functional and balanced cognitions. These in turn improve mood and result in less avoidance and withdrawal.

Cognitive biases generate unpleasant emotions and affect how we behave.

▶ The cognitive model

Based largely on the work of Beck, the way in which dysfunctional cognitive processes are acquired, activated, and effect behaviour and emotions is summarised diagrammatically in the model below.

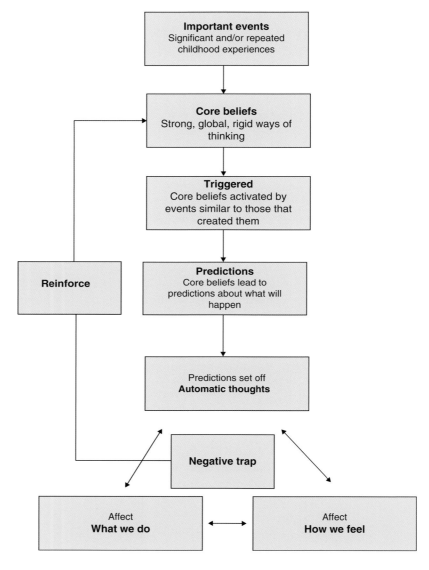

Early experiences and parenting are hypothesised to lead to the development of fairly fixed and rigid ways of thinking, i.e. core beliefs/schemas. These beliefs/schemas are activated by events similar to the ones that established them and form a framework for perceiving the world. New information and experiences are assessed against these core beliefs/schemas and lead to predictions about what will happen (i.e. assumptions). For example, a core belief such as 'I am a failure' may be activated by an important event such as 'taking exams'. This may result in an assumption such as 'No matter how hard I work I will never get a good mark'. Beliefs and assumptions produce a stream of automatic thoughts. These are related to the person ('I must be stupid'), their performance ('I can't do this'), and the future ('I'll never pass these exams'). These automatic thoughts effect how we feel (e.g. anxious and unhappy) and what we do (e.g. stop revising and not motivated), and in turn strengthen the original belief that 'I am a failure'.

In addition to understanding the different levels of cognitions, CBT also pays attention to their specific content and the nature of the processing deficits and biases. There is an assumption of specificity, i.e. that specific processing deficits and biases are associated with particular emotional problems. However, they are not mutually exclusive, although there are some general trends (Garber and Weersing 2010). In general, young people who are anxious tend to have cognitions and biases towards the future and personal threat, danger, vulnerability, and inability to cope (Schniering and Rapee 2004; Muris and Field 2008). Depression tends to be related to cognitions concerning loss, deprivation, and personal failure with rumination increasing feelings of hopelessness (Kendall, Stark, and Adam 1990; Leitenberg, Yost, and Carroll-Wilson 1986; Rehm and Carter 1990). Aggressive young people tend to perceive more aggressive intent in ambiguous situations, selectively attend to fewer cues when making decisions about the intent of another person's behaviour, and generate fewer verbal solutions to problems (Dodge 1985; Lochman, White, and Wayland 1991; Perry, Perry, and Rasmussen 1986).

Interventions addressing cognitive distortions are concerned with increasing the young person's awareness of biased and unhelpful cognitions, beliefs, and schemas and, facilitating their understanding of the effects of these upon behaviour and emotions. Programmes typically involve some form of self-monitoring, identification of maladaptive cognitions, thought testing, and cognitive restructuring.

Challenging and changing cognitions can improve mood.

An extension of this work, Schema-Focused Therapy, was developed by Young (1994) for those who failed to respond or relapsed following traditional CBT. Schema-Focused Therapy was based on the recognition that some people seem to develop life-long self-defeating patterns of behaviour that are repeated throughout life. Young proposed that this was the result of early maladaptive schemas, strong and rigid ways of thinking that are formed during childhood and which are resistant to change. These are associated with particular trauma and parenting styles and develop if the basic emotional needs of the child are not met. Evidence to support the presence of 15 primary schemas has been reported (Schmidt et al. 1995) with subsequent research identifying the presence of cognitive schemas in adolescents and children as young as eight (Rijkeboer and Boo 2010; Stallard 2007; Stallard and Rayner 2005). Schema-Focused Therapy pays greater attention to the past and understanding these lifelong patterns rather than upon specific situations and events.

Maladaptive cognitive schema/beliefs develop during childhood.

▶ Third wave: acceptance, compassion, and mindfulness

Whilst the second wave Cognitive Therapies have proven very effective they do not work for everyone. Some people do not find the process of actively challenging and re-appraising specific cognitions easy or acceptable. Similarly, a number of studies have highlighted that changes in cognitions are not necessarily related to improved emotional well-being. Changes occur without directly and explicitly challenging the content of cognitions. This led to a third wave of CBTs which focus on changing the nature of the relationship between the individual and their own internal events rather than actively changing the content of their cognitions. This is achieved through the development and integration of skills that promote health and well-being into everyday life.

> Grounded in an empirical, principle-focused approach, the third wave of behavioral and cognitive therapy is particularly sensitive to the context and functions of psychological phenomena, not just their form, and thus tends to emphasise contextual and experiential change strategies in addition to more direct and didactic ones. (Hayes 2004)

> Thoughts and feelings are ongoing events, not expressions of reality.

ACT was developed by Stephen Hayes and uses acceptance and mindfulness strategies to confront, experience, and accept unpleasant thoughts and feelings (Hayes, Strosahl, and Wilson 1999; Hayes et al. 2006). Through this process young people learn to accept that they can live with and tolerate unpleasant experiences, emotions, and thoughts rather than viewing them as intolerable events and which they need to change.

ACT utilises six core psychological processes to develop psychological flexibility, i.e. the ability to connect with the present moment and inner experiences without defence. The first, acceptance, involves actively embracing inner experiences which are happening here and now as ongoing inner experiences. Cognitive defusion reduces the impact of these experiences by changing the context in which they occur. The natural tendency to rectify thoughts and emotions is countered by learning to accept them as simply thoughts and feelings. The third process promotes personal awareness of the here and now as attention is focused without judgement on internal and external events as they occur through the use of mindfulness-based techniques. Fourth, the individual is helped to develop their self-image with the fifth process focusing upon identifying those aspects of life which are personally important. These values provide an ongoing framework for motivating and guiding future behaviour. Finally, committed action is where the person pursues their values, whilst practicing acceptance, cognitive defusion, and being present.

> Accept thoughts and feelings that occur rather than trying to change or eliminate them.

CFT attempts to understand how our minds work and arose from observations that people with high levels of self-criticism and shame find it hard to be kind to themselves. Gilbert (2014) suggested that this is caused by an imbalance in basic emotional evolutionary systems designed to protect, motivate, and sooth. These basic systems (old brain) hijack our more recently developed meta-cognitive systems (new brain) which allow us to imagine, reason, and ruminate. The old brain's protection and drive systems dominate as our cognitive processes are drawn to, and increase our awareness of, threat. Our ability to sooth ourselves by suppressing unpleasant emotions or stimulating positive emotions is impaired, resulting in people finding it difficult to feel safe or content with themselves.

Compassion-focused therapy focuses on helping to feel safe, to develop self-soothing, and to replace self-criticism with self-kindness (Gilbert 2007). This is achieved through compassionate mind training which creates feelings of warmth and kindness as we develop a more soothing approach. Compassionate attention helps us to be mindful of our thoughts and emotions and to focus on our strengths, positive skills, and acts of kindness. Compassionate reasoning develops more balanced, kinder, alternative thinking where self-criticism is replaced with a compassionate approach. Compassionate behaviour encourages us to behave in helpful ways such as facing frightening events or being kind to ourselves. Compassionate imagery helps to create our positive self-image and to promote the values that are important to us whilst compassionate feeling helps to notice and experience acts of kindness from others.

> Lean to look after yourself and to be kind and compassionate.

Another recent development is Dialectical Behaviour Therapy (DBT). This was developed by Marsha Linehan to change patterns of behaviour that are unhelpful and destructive (Linehan 1993). It is based on the premise that psychological problems result from deficits in emotional regulation skills. This is addressed by increasing awareness of triggers that lead to states of high emotion and developing a range of skills to cope with stress, regulate emotions, and improve relationships.

Dialectics assumes that everything is composed of opposites and that both acceptance and change are necessary requirements to improve emotional regulation and distress tolerance. Thus, accepting that distressing events, thoughts, and feelings occur, but changing how these are responded to. To achieve this, DBT develops skills in the core areas of mindfulness, distress tolerance, emotion regulation, and interpersonal effectiveness (Koerner 2012). Mindfulness helps the individual to non-judgementally observe, accept, and tolerate powerful unpleasant emotions rather than being overwhelmed by them. This helps to make wise decisions about how to respond and tolerate distress through the use of a range of techniques including distraction and self-soothing. The idea is to learn to tolerate distress rather than trying to change situations or events that cause it. Emotional regulation is developed through promoting greater awareness of emotional signals, triggering events, and problems-solving. The final area is the developing of interpersonal effectiveness skills and strategies for being assertive and coping with interpersonal conflict.

> Accept and tolerate distress, manage emotions, and improve interpersonal effectiveness.

Finally, mindfulness-based CBT (MBCT) was developed by Zindel Segal, Mark Williams, and John Teasdale and is based on work pioneered by Jon Kabat-Zinn. Buddhist meditation techniques are used to develop cognitive awareness by actively focusing attention on the present moment. It involves curious non-judgemental observation and acceptance of thoughts and feelings in which cognitions and emotions are experienced as ongoing and passing mental events. Through increased awareness, the individual is better able to deal with their thoughts and feelings. The focus is not on changing the content of the thoughts, but to experience them as internal events separated from the self and to accept them in a non-judgemental way (Segal, Williams, and Teasdale 2002).

> Focus attention on the present moment in a curious, non-judgemental way.

▶ Core characteristics of CBT

Although CBT is an umbrella term to describe a family of different interventions, they nonetheless share a number of core features.

CBT is theoretically determined

CBT is based upon empirically testable models. Strong theoretical models provide the rationale for CBT, i.e. that cognitions are associated with emotional problems and inform the content of the intervention, i.e. change the nature of the cognitions or our relationship with them. CBT therefore provides a cohesive and rational intervention and is not simply a collection of disparate techniques.

CBT is based on a collaborative model

A key feature of CBT is the collaborative process by which it occurs. The young person has an active role with regard to identifying their goals, setting targets, experimenting, practicing, and monitoring their performance. The approach is designed to facilitate greater and more effective self-control, with the therapist providing a supportive framework within which this can occur. The role of the therapist is to develop a partnership in which the young person is empowered to develop a better understanding of their problems and to discover alternative ways of thinking and behaving.

CBT is time-limited

It is often brief and usually time-limited, consisting of no more than 16 sessions, and in many cases, far fewer than this. The brief nature of the intervention promotes independence and encourages self-help. This model is readily applicable to work with young people, for whom the typical period of intervention is considerably shorter than that with adults.

CBT is objective and structured

It is a structured and objective approach that guides the young person through a process of assessment, problem formulation, intervention, monitoring, and evaluation. The goals and targets of the intervention are explicitly defined and regularly reviewed. There is an emphasis on quantification and the use of ratings (e.g. the frequency of inappropriate behaviour, strength of belief in thoughts, or degree of distress experienced). Regular monitoring and reviewing provide a way of assessing progress by comparing current performance against baseline assessments.

CBT has a here-and-now focus

CBT interventions focus upon the present, dealing with current problems and difficulties. They do not seek to 'uncover unconscious early trauma or biological, neurological, and genetic contributions to psychological dysfunction, but instead strives to build a new, more adaptive way to process the world' (Kendall and Panichelli-Mindel 1995). This approach has high-face validity for young people, who may be more interested in and motivated to address real time, here-and-now issues, rather than understanding their origins.

CBT is based on a process of guided self-discovery and experimentation

It is an active process that encourages self-questioning and the development and practice of new skills. Young people are not simply passive recipients of therapist's advice or observations but are encouraged to observe and learn through a process of experimentation. The link between thoughts and feelings is investigated and alternative ways of changing the content or nature of our relationship with our thoughts explored.

CBT is a skill-based approach

CBT provides a practical, skills-based approach to learn alternative patterns of thinking and behaviour. Young people are encouraged to practice skills and ideas that are discussed during therapy sessions in their everyday life, with home practice tasks being a core element of many programmes. These provide opportunities to identify what is helpful and how potential problems can be resolved.

CBT is theoretically determined.

It is based on a model of active collaboration.

It is brief and time limited.

It is objective and structured.

It focuses on current problems.

It encourages self-discovery and experimentation.

It advocates a skills-based learning approach.

▶ The goal of cognitive behaviour therapy

The overall purpose of CBT is to improve current well-being, resilience, and future coping. This is achieved through developing increased self-awareness, improved self-control, and enhancing personal efficacy through the promotion of helpful cognitive and behavioural skills. The process of CBT moves the young person from a dysfunctional to a more functional cycle as illustrated below.

Dysfunctional cycle

Thoughts
Overly negative
Self-critical and judgemental
Selective and biased

Behaviour
Avoid
Give up
Inappropriate
Unhelpful

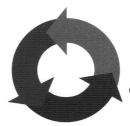

Feelings
Unpleasant
Anxious
Depressed
Angry
Out of control

Functional cycle

Thoughts
More positive and balanced
Acknowledge success and strengths
Accepting and non-judgemental

Behaviour
Confront
Try
Appropriate
Helpful

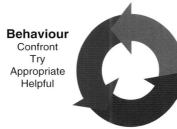

Feelings
Pleasant
Relaxed
Happy
Calm
In control

CBT helps to reduce the negative effect of what people think (cognitions) on how they feel (emotions), and what they do (behaviour). This is achieved by either actively focusing on the content of the young person's cognitions or by changing the nature of their relationship with them.

- If focusing on content, the young person is encouraged to observe and identify common dysfunctional thoughts and beliefs that are predominantly negative, biased, and self-critical. Through a process of self-monitoring, education, and experimentation, these are tested and replaced by more balanced and functional cognitions that acknowledge strengths and success.

- If focusing on their relationship with their cognitions, the young person is encouraged to stand back from their thoughts and to observe them in a curious, non-judgemental way as passing cognitive activity. Mindfulness maintains attention on the here and now with the young person being encouraged to accept themselves and the events that occur.

▶ The core components of CBT

CBT includes a range of techniques and strategies that can be used in different sequences and permutations. This flexibility allows interventions to be tailored towards particular problems and the needs of the young person rather than being delivered in a standardised cook book approach. Similarly, the wealth of techniques means that CBT can be used for prevention to enhance coping and resilience as well as an intervention to reduce psychological distress.

Although the primary focus of second wave (i.e. test and challenge the content of cognitions and processes) and third wave (i.e. change the nature of the relationship with our thoughts) CBT differ, embedded within these approaches are a number of different skills and techniques.

Psycho-education

A basic component of all cognitive behavioural programmes involves education about CBT and the link *between thoughts, feelings, and behaviour*. The process involves developing a clear and shared understanding of the relationship between how people think, how they feel, and what they do. In addition, the collaborative process of CBT and the active role of practice and experimentation are stressed.

Values, goals, and targets

CBT may involve identifying important *personal values*. These help to maintain focus on the future and act as a framework for motivating and guiding behaviour towards their achievement.

Goal setting is an inherent part of all cognitive behaviour programmes. The *overall goals* of therapy are mutually agreed and defined in ways that can be objectively assessed. The transfer of skills from therapy sessions to everyday life is encouraged by the systematic use of *assignment tasks* where new skills are practiced in real-life settings. The achievement of *specified targets* is regularly reviewed and provides an overview of progress.

Acceptance and acknowledgement of strengths

CBT helps the individual to see the complete picture so that their *strengths and achievements* are recognised and acknowledged. Personal strengths can be empowering and can be used to cope with future challenges and problems. *Acceptance* is also emphasised so that rather than constantly trying to change things which are beyond their control these are accepted for what they are.

Thought monitoring

A key task is to develop a better understanding of common cognitions which is achieved through observing and monitoring cognitions and patterns of thinking. Thought monitoring could focus on the specific content of *core beliefs, negative automatic thoughts, or dysfunctional assumptions* to identify those that produce strong emotional reactions or are overly negative or self-critical. Alternatively, *observation* could be encouraged whereby the young person is helped to develop an understanding of the effect of their cognitions on their emotions.

Identification of cognitive distortions and deficits

The process of thought monitoring provides an opportunity to identify common *negative or unhelpful cognitions, beliefs, or assumptions*. In turn this results in increased awareness of the nature and type of *cognitive distortions* (e.g. magnification and focusing upon the negative), *cognitive deficits* (e.g. misinterpretation of others cues as negative and limited range of problem-solving skills) and the effect of these upon mood and behaviour.

Thought evaluation and developing alternative cognitive processes

The identification of dysfunctional cognitive processes leads to the systematic *testing and evaluating of these assumptions and beliefs* and the learning of alternative cognitive skills. The development of a process of *balanced thinking* or *cognitive restructuring* is encouraged. This may involve a process of looking for new information, thinking from another persons' perspective, or looking for contradictory evidence, which may result in dysfunctional cognitions, being revised.

The evaluation provides an opportunity to develop alternative, *more balanced and functional* cognitions, which recognise difficulties but acknowledge strengths and success.

Development of new cognitive skills

CBT involves the development of new cognitive skills such as *distraction* where attention is focused away from anxiety-increasing stimuli towards more neutral tasks. Cognitive coping can be enhanced through the use of *positive self-talk and self-instructional training* with *consequential thinking and problem-solving skills* helping to develop alternative ways of thinking through challenges.

Mindfulness

In addition, CBT may develop cognitive skills such as *mindfulness* where attention is focused non-judgementally on the present moment. Rather than reacting to or attempting to change what we think or how we feel mindfulness helps to develop curious observation of our internal processes. This in turn reduces negative cognitive rehearsal of future events and rumination about past events.

Affective education

Many programmes involve emotional education designed to *identify and distinguish core emotions* such as anger, anxiety, or unhappiness. Programmes may focus upon the *physiological changes* associated with these emotions (e.g. dry mouth, sweaty hands, and increased heart rate) in order to facilitate a greater awareness of the young person's unique expression of each core emotion.

Affective monitoring

The monitoring of strong or dominant emotions can help identify *times, places, activities, or thoughts* that are associated with both pleasant and unpleasant feelings. *Scales* are used to rate the intensity of emotion both during real-life situations and treatment sessions and provide an objective way of monitoring performance and assessing change.

Affective management

New emotional management skills are developed to help *tolerate distress* and/or manage emotions more effectively. This may involve techniques such as *progressive muscle relaxation, controlled breathing, calming imagery, self-soothing,* or *distraction.*

Greater awareness of the individual's unique emotional pattern can lead to the development of *preventative strategies.* An awareness of the anger build up may, for example, enable a young person to stop the emotional progression at an earlier stage and prevent aggressive outbursts. Similarly the adoption of *helpful habits* throughout everyday life can help to prevent future problems occurring.

Activity monitoring

This can be used to promote awareness of the link between *what we do and how we feel and behave.* This helps to develop a better understanding of what we do and how some activities or events are associated with different feelings and ways of thinking.

Behaviour activation

Activity monitoring can lead to *behavioural activation* whereby the individual is encouraged to become more active. This may involve *increasing activities* that create enjoyment, involve others, produce a sense of achievement or encourage physical activity. Activity can have a positive effect upon mood.

Activity rescheduling

Engagement in activities that create more pleasant emotions can also be encouraged by *activity rescheduling*. This involves rescheduling positive mood-lifting activities to occur at those days or times that are currently associated with strong unpleasant emotions.

Skills development

A structured *problem-solving* process can provide a useful framework for confronting and dealing with challenges rather than putting decisions off or avoiding them. A number of CBT interventions also focus on the development of *interpersonal effectiveness* by enhancing skills such as conflict resolution, assertiveness, and developing and maintaining friendships.

Behavioural experiments

CBT is based upon a process of guided discovery during which assumptions and thoughts are challenged and tested. A powerful way to do this is to objectively check things out by setting up *behavioural experiments*. These can help to test whether predictions and thoughts are always right, to discover alternative explanations for events, or what might happen if things were done differently.

Fear hierarchy and exposure

A core aim of CBT programmes is to encourage the young person to face and learn to cope with challenging situations or events. This can be achieved through a process of *graduated exposure* where problems are defined, the overall task broken into smaller steps, and then each is ranked in a hierarchy of ascending difficulty. Starting with the least difficult, the young person is exposed to each step of the *hierarchy*, either in vivo or imagination. Once successfully completed, they move to the next step, progressing through the hierarchy until the problem has been mastered.

Role play, modelling, exposure, and rehearsal

The learning of new skills and behaviours can be achieved in a variety of ways. *Role-play* provides an opportunity to practice dealing with difficult or challenging situations such as coping with teasing. Role-play enables positive skills to be identified and alternative solutions or new skills highlighted. A process of *skills enhancement* can facilitate the process of acquiring new skills and behaviours. Observing others *model appropriate behaviour* or skills can then result in new behaviour being *rehearsed* in imagination before being *practiced in real life* through *exposure* tasks.

Self-reinforcement and reward

A cornerstone of all CBT programmes is *positive reinforcement* and acknowledgement of effort. We need to care for ourselves and to value what we do. This could take the form of *self-reinforcement*, for example, cognitively (e.g. 'Well done, I coped well with that situation'), materially (e.g. purchasing a special CD), or by activities (e.g. special relaxing bath). Reinforcement should be based on effort and attempting to do things rather than upon the achievement of a successful outcome.

   The above provides the clinician with a rich tool box of CBT techniques that can be used flexibly with young people. These are summarised in The clinician's toolbox.

CBT provides a rich toolbox of techniques and ideas that can be flexibly used to increase self-awareness, improve self-control, and enhance personal efficacy through the promotion of helpful cognitive, emotional, and behavioural skills.

▶ The clinician's toolbox

Psycho-education
Understand the link between thoughts, feelings, and behaviour

Values, goals, and targets
Identify personal values, agree goals, and targets

Acceptance and acknowledgement of strengths
Recognise positives and strengths and accepting who you are

Cognitions

Thought monitoring
Negative automatic thoughts
Core beliefs/schema
Dysfunctional assumptions

Identification of cognitive distortions and deficits
Common dysfunctional cognitions, assumptions and beliefs
Patterns of cognitive distortions
Cognitive deficits

Thought evaluation
Testing and evaluating cognitions
Cognitive restructuring
Development of alternative, balanced thinking

Development of new cognitive skills
Distraction, positive and coping self-talk
Self-instructional training, consequential thinking

Mindfulness
Curious and non-judgemental observation

Behaviour ——————————— Emotions

Activity monitoring
Link activity, thoughts and feelings

Behavioural activation
Increase mood lifting activity

Activity rescheduling
Timetable activities

Skills development
Problem solving and interpersonal effectiveness

Behavioural experiments
Test predictions/assumptions
Discover new meanings

Fear hierarchy and exposure
Face challenges in a graded way

Affective education
Distinguish between core emotions
Identify physiological bodily symptoms

Affective monitoring
Link feelings with thoughts and behaviour
Scales to rate intensity

Affective management
Relaxation, self-soothing, mind games,
imagery, controlled breathing

Self-reinforcement
Take care of yourself and reward yourself

CHAPTER TWO

The process of cognitive behaviour therapy

Cognitive behaviour therapy (CBT) is founded on a guiding principle of collaborative empiricism whereby the clinician and young person work together to discover new understandings and ways of coping. This is achieved through a process of guided discovery where the young person is encouraged to experiment and to be open and curious about their cognitions. This helps the young person to develop a new relationship with their cognitions and to question the meanings they ascribe to events. The process is positive and empowering as the young person discovers new cognitive skills and processes.

▶ Therapeutic process

CBT occurs within the context of a strong therapeutic relationship built upon warmth, empathy, and understanding (Beck et al. 1979). The relationship is open, honest, and non-judgemental with the young person and clinician actively working together.

A number of specific aspects of the therapeutic relationship have been identified as important. Creed and Kendall (2005) noted the significance of collaboration, where the young person and clinician work together as a team, with mutually agreed goals, and where the young person is actively involved in the intervention. Clinician flexibility and creativity are also important. This involves making sessions engaging and active through presenting ideas and concepts in multiple formats such as games and role plays, appropriately adapted to the interests of the young person (Chu and Kendall 2009). Similarly, clinicians who are warm, positive, and empathic develop better relationships with young people than those who are aloof or patronising or push them to talk about uncomfortable emotions (Russell, Shirk, and Jungbluth 2008). Establishing a good therapeutic relationship is associated with better engagement, increased motivation, and superior outcomes (Chiu et al. 2009; McLeod and Weisz 2005; Shirk and Karver 2003; Karver et al. 2006; McLeod 2011).

Another aspect of the therapeutic process which is important for CBT is the development of collaborative inquiry where young people 'become scientific investigators of their own thinking' (Beck and Dozois 2011, p. 400). The promotion of a reflective and investigative approach requires careful attention since young people are often more familiar with being provided with information and answers rather than discovering their own solutions. Finally, the need to adapt CBT to the developmental level of the young person has been emphasised by many writers (Stallard 2003; Friedberg and McClure 2015) and has been reflected in different versions of CBT programmes for children and adolescents (Barrett 2005a,b). This requires CBT to be pitched at a level which is consistent with the young person's cognitive, emotional, verbal, and reasoning ability.

Thinking Good, Feeling Better: A Cognitive Behavioural Therapy Workbook for Adolescents and Young Adults, First Edition.
Paul Stallard.
© 2019 John Wiley & Sons Ltd. Published 2019 by John Wiley & Sons Ltd.
Companion website: www.wiley.com/go/thinkinggood

Stallard (2005) has defined the key elements of the therapeutic process with young people by the acronym **PRECISE**.

P – Partnership: This emphasises the collaborative nature of CBT and the importance of the therapeutic partnership whereby the young person has an active role in securing change.

R – Right developmental level: The clinician carefully attends to the young person's developmental level in order to ensure that the intervention is consistent with their cognitive, linguistic, memory, and perspective-taking abilities. Pitching the intervention too high will result in the young person failing to understand the model whilst pitching it too low may be perceived as patronising.

E – Empathy: Focuses on developing and maintaining a relationship based on warmth, genuine concern, and respect. This is fostered through important interpersonal skills such as active listening, reflection, and summaries.

C – Creativity: Identifies the need to be flexible and creative in conveying the concepts of CBT in ways that match the young person's interests and experiences.

I – Investigation: A curious, open, and inquisitive approach is encouraged where thoughts, feelings, and behaviours are subject to objective evaluation through Socratic dialogues and behavioural experiments.

S – Self-efficacy: The process should encourage self-reflection and discovery. This empowers the young person to develop a better understanding of their cognitions and to discover ways in which these can be processed in more helpful ways

E – Engagement and enjoyment: Finally, the process should be enjoyable and engaging so that the young person's interest, commitment, and motivation are maintained.

> CBT is based on a strong empathic relationship which encourages openness, curiosity, and self-discovery.

▶ Phases of CBT

The clinician will guide the young person though a number of phases each with a different primary aim. The length of time spent in each phase will vary according to the young person's needs.

Relationship building and engagement

Thus is the initial phase of CBT where the primary focus is upon developing the therapeutic partnership and engaging the young person in the process of change. This phase is particularly important since young people rarely seek help in their own right. Typically, they are identified by others and as such may not recognise or acknowledge any problems and may initially appear unmotivated or disinterested (McLeod and Weisz 2005; Creed and Kendall 2005; Shirk and Karver 2003).

Engagement can be developed through interpersonal skills such as active listening and empathy. Active listening conveys interest and demonstrates that the clinician respects and understands the young person whilst empathy shows that they understand how they feel. The relationship is strengthened through an open and non-judgemental stance where the young person's difficulties and potential ambivalence are validated and acknowledged.

The young person's motivation to engage in CBT can be enhanced by focusing on how they would like their life to be different and the targets they would like to achieve. The miracle question from solution-focused brief therapy can help the young person to focus on the future rather than remaining stuck with their problems in the present moment (de Shazer 1985). The miracle question asks the young person to think how and what would be different if they no longer had a problem:

> Imagine that whilst you slept tonight a miracle happened and all your problems were sorted. When you awake tomorrow, what would you notice that would tell you that life had suddenly got better?

Once some degree of commitment to securing change is established, clear goals need to be agreed and defined. The SMART acronym helps to ensure that goals are specific, measurable, achievable, relevant, and timely. A good goal should be specific, e.g. 'to call my friend Joe twice per week' rather than general and vague 'to be more sociable'. When goals are specific, it is easier to know what needs to be achieved whilst establishing concrete criteria, e.g. 'twice per week' allows the young person to objectively measure their progress. Motivation will be enhanced by successful achievement of meaningful goals. Goals should not be so large that they are difficult to achieve and should relate to relevant and important aspects of the young person's life. Finally, to maintain motivation, goals need to be achieved within a realistic time frame.

Engaging and motivating the young person is a pre-requisite to the subsequent stages of CBT. The therapist therefore presents as open, understanding, positive, and hopeful as they elicit commitment from the young person to 'give it a try'.

Psycho-education

Psycho-education involves providing the young person with information and primarily focuses upon three main areas.

First, the young person is socialised into the process of CBT and in particular the concept of collaborative empiricism. The collaborative nature of the relationship is explained with the clinician providing a structure and framework for the young person to use to reflect on their own experiences. The active role of the young person in testing ideas and undertaking experiments to discover what happens and works for them is highlighted. The need to suspend judgement and to adopt an open and curious approach is stressed and the importance of the young person's contributions highlighted.

Second, the young person is socialised into the cognitive model. Information is provided about the link between events, thoughts, feelings, and behaviours. The central role of cognitions in determining how they feel and what they do is stressed. This provides the rationale for CBT, i.e. to understand their thoughts and to change the relationship with them by either questioning or accepting them. Through the development of more helpful cognitive processes, the young person will feel better and be able to confront challenging situations and deal with their problems. Finally, the effectiveness of CBT in alleviating many emotional problems is highlighted. The clinician remains optimistic and hopeful, but is unable to guarantee that CBT is always successful or suits everyone.

These first two aspects of psycho-education occur during the initial stages of the intervention, although they will be regularly revisited during the course of the intervention. Indeed, the underling cognitive model provides the rationale for the intervention and helps to explain the focus of the work.

In addition to the above, psycho-education about specific emotional problems will also be required. Anxious young people, for example, may require information about the flight-fight response and some of the physiological bodily changes that accompany anxiety. Similarly, information about low mood and depression and the physiological changes in eating, sleeping, concentration, and social withdrawal can help young people to make sense of their experience. Psycho-education can be undertaken collaboratively by encouraging the young person to use the Internet to research specific questions.

Promoting self-awareness and understanding

During this phase, the young person is encouraged to become aware of their own cognitions, emotions, and behaviours and to use the CBT framework to understand the relationship between them. This can be achieved through self-monitoring where diaries and records are used to identify situations or events that the young person finds difficult. For example, they could be helped to become more aware of their thoughts by watching out for the 'hot thoughts' that produce a strong emotional reaction. Diaries and computer logs can help to identify and understand different types of cognitions (helpful and unhelpful thoughts), processing biases (thinking traps), and common dysfunctional cognitions.

Self-understanding can also be developed through behavioural experiments in which the young person objectively tests their cognitions. Behavioural experiments can be used to test whether their beliefs or assumptions are always true or to discover what might happen if they behaved differently. Another type of experiment, surveys, can help to discover new information which can be used by the young person to re-assess the understandings and meanings they assign to events.

Every experiment provides an opportunity for self-reflection and the development of greater insight and understanding. An exposure task whereby the young person confronts a feared situation might help to discover that anxiety reduces over time. Becoming busy through behavioural activation might help a depressed young person understand that they can do something to make themselves feel better.

Finally, self-awareness can lead to the adoption of a new approach to life. Mindfulness, for example, can help to increase awareness of thoughts and emotions. Learning to observe these in a non-judgemental way can help young people understand them as passing experiences which they do not need to react to or argue with.

Enhancing skills and development

In addition to promoting self-understanding and awareness, CBT also develops new cognitive, emotional and behavioural skills. In terms of cognitions, young people might develop new skills to challenge specific cognitions or processing biases. Alternatively, they might learn to be mindful of their cognitions and to accept them as passing thoughts rather than as evidence of reality. Rather than being negative and self-critical young people can learn to value themselves for who they are. To accept and forgive their mistakes and to speak to themselves in a kinder way as they develop an alternative approach to life.

Emotional skills may lead to the better management of unpleasant emotions. A tool box of emotional skills may be developed such as relaxation training, controlled breathing, or calming imagery. Activity rescheduling may be used to reduce the intensity or frequency of unpleasant emotions and self-soothing techniques developed to help face and tolerate distress.

In terms of behaviour, interventions may involve developing more adaptive behaviours in which problem-solving, social, and personal effectiveness skills such as assertion and negotiation are enhanced. This may involve techniques such as role play, observational exercises, graded exposure, behavioural activation, or response prevention. Finally, the young person is encouraged to celebrate their achievements.

Consolidation

Once learned, the new skills need to be practiced and integrated into the young person's everyday repertoire.

Whilst skills might be helpful when used in a session, they need to be tested under real-life conditions. This is particularly important during the latter stages of the intervention as the young person develops a different approach to everyday life. This can be achieved through the use of out-of-session tasks which are agreed with the young person. Through practice, the young person learns to sharpen their new skills and to respond differently to situations.

There will be a natural tendency to slip back into old habits and so clearly defined times to practice need to be encouraged. This can be facilitated through the use of visual and audio prompts. A piece of tape on a tooth brush can serve as a prompt to be mindful or an alarm on a phone as a prompt to look for acts of kindness.

Finally, in order to sustain the use of these new skills, they need to be integrated into the young person's daily routine. Explore ways in which the use of skills can be associated with everyday events such as dressing, eating, or getting into bed.

Relapse prevention

The final phase is relapse prevention where the young person is encouraged to reflect on those aspects of the intervention that have been helpful, to prepare for possible relapse, and to develop a contingency plan in case problems re-emerge.

The development of a 'keeping well' plan helps the young person to reflect on what they have discovered and the skills they have found useful. They are prepared to expect setbacks. These are viewed as normal and temporary rather than a return of their old problems or evidence that their skills are no longer effective. They are helped to identify future situations that could potentially be difficult and to become aware of the warning signs that might suggest that they are slipping back into their old habits. They are encouraged to stay positive and to be kind to themselves, accepting that things will go wrong and that unkind things happen. Finally, they are helped to plan what to do if they become stuck in their old habits and when and how to seek help.

> CBT involves relationship building and engagement, psycho-education, self-awareness and understanding, skill development and enhancement, and consolidation and relapse prevention.

▶ Adapting CBT for young people

The evidence base for CBT has been established through many randomised controlled trials with young people aged 7–25 years of age. Many of the early studies were based on the premise that adolescents had sufficiently developed linguistic, cognitive, emotional, and social perspective skills to engage in CBT. Programmes were often downward extensions of those developed for adults and were heavily reliant on verbal discussion. Young people were viewed as 'small adults' possessing the fully developed skills expected in adulthood. This position has been challenged with a greater awareness of the developmental changes during childhood and adolescence now informing the way CBT is adapted for young people (Holmbeck et al. 2006; Sauter, Heyne, and Westenberg 2009).

Adolescence is a stage of rapid physical and psychological development that marks the transition from childhood to adulthood. It is the stage where young people develop their own self-identity, form strong opinions, and develop their own moral and ethical values. Young people become more autonomous as they seek independence and establish deeper and more meaningful relationships with their peers. The increased independence and ability to make decisions will result in experimentation and risk-taking.

In terms of cognitive development, young people become more able to engage in abstract thinking and to understand multiple perspectives as linguistic, reasoning, metacognition, and social perspective-taking skills develop. Metacognition is the ability to think about one's own thinking, whilst social perspective taking is the ability to view events from the perspective of another. Given the wide age range covered by adolescence, it cannot be assumed that these skills are fully developed in all young people. Clinicians need to ensure that CBT is adapted to the adolescents abilities not their physical appearance and to remain aware that not all adolescents can engage in all cognitive techniques (Sauter, Heyne, and Westenberg 2009). However, there is no simple way of assessing cognitive development across different cognitive sub-domains (Holmbeck et al. 2006). Furthermore, these are not essential prerequisites for undertaking CBT with young people. Given that CBT is effective with children with more limited cognitive skills, it is clear that interventions can be successful if carefully adjusted to the capacities of the young person. In so doing, the clinician will need to consider a number of factors including the following.

Cognitive vs behavioural focus

An optimum balance between cognitive and behavioural techniques needs to be established. As a general rule, if a young person finds it difficult to engage in cognitive techniques, then a greater emphasis should be placed on behavioural methods (Friedberg and McClure 2015; Stallard 2009). These are more concrete activities where the young person's cognitions are explored through 'doing' behavioural experiments rather than through cognitive debate and discussion. Other young people may have well-developed cognitive capacities and find complex metacognitive work more engaging and helpful. They might find simpler techniques which focus on developing positive or helpful thinking (i.e. self-talk) as simplistic and patronising.

Therapeutic partnership

CBT is based on a therapeutic relationship where the young person and clinician are equal partners. This is important, but it needs to be recognised that there is an inherent power imbalance between the clinician and young person. It is therefore important that the nature of the partnership is made explicit at the start of CBT; otherwise, the young person will expect the clinician to be active and to take a lead role.

Objective empiricism should be promoted, and the clinician should explicitly acknowledge that they do not have the solutions, but that they will work with the young person to discover what works for them. The notion of learning together should be highlighted, and the clinician should be mindful of ways in which the young person's active and leading role can be promoted. This can be promoted in a number of ways including inviting the young person to take a lead role in establishing goals, determining the agenda, order, and content of sessions (Stallard 2013). At other times, the young person may be less mature and benefit from more direct guidance from the clinician (Friedberg and McClure 2015).

Language

Third, the use of language should be considered to ensure that it is pitched at the right level for the young person. This can be achieved by employing the young person's own language to describe events. For example, a young person may talk about 'over-thinking' as a way of explaining cognitive rumination or rehearsal or talk about 'tuning out' as they describe how they learn not to argue with their thoughts. The exact meaning of the words needs to be established, but can then be used as a shared way of talking about concepts.

The clinician also needs to be careful in their use of terminology, for example, describing practice tasks as homework. Although practice is an important part of CBT, the term homework may have negative connotations for young people. Homework often implies that young person has been given (rather than agreed) a task. It is usually something they would not chose to do, and as such is somewhat at odds with the notion of guided discovery that is central to CBT. Finally, homework is often marked and typically involves some form of grading, whilst in CBT the goal is often discovery and reflection. An alternative might be to talk about out-of-session assignments or practice.

Metaphors provide a very helpful way of relating abstract concepts to concrete events familiar to the young person. For example, metaphors can be used to describe abstract cognitive processing biases such as catastrophisation or selective abstraction as disaster thinking or negative glasses. Automatic thoughts can be conceptualised as computer spam or 'pop-ups' and the metaphor developed to help young people develop a robust firewall.

Dichotomous thinking

The egotistical and categorical thinking so commonly encountered during adolescence can interfere with the process of CBT. Egotistical adolescents may be unable to recognise another perspective and therefore unable to consider alternative views. Similarly, 'all or nothing' thinking is common with young people and is often reflected in dramatic swings from session to session. On one occasion, an adolescent may present as depressed or anxious, whilst by the next, they are happy or relaxed.

Rating scales are a useful way of challenging dichotomous thinking and help the young person to recognise that there are a range of options between their two extreme anchor points. This may require some degree of education and could involve the young person rating or ordering a series of events along a particular dimension. Scales can be used to rate the intensity of feelings, belief in thoughts, degree of responsibility, or blame.

Finally, Belsher and Wilkes (1993), highlight the importance of the language used by the clinician. Asking what would be 'good' or 'bad' suggests a dichotomous categorisation, whereas 'better' or 'worse' conveys the impression of a graded continuum.

Verbal vs non-verbal materials

Both verbal and non-verbal methods can be used with young people to explain the ideas and concepts of CBT. Some young people may have very good linguistic skills and enjoy abstract debate and reasoning. They may be very talkative and feel comfortable discussing themselves and their problems and engage fully in a verbal approach.

Others may feel embarrassed taking to a clinician and may find non-verbal methods easier to engage with. These could involve the use of whiteboards, cartoons, thought bubbles, or story boards to explain the thoughts and feelings that might accompany particular events. Diagrams summarising the CBT model can be very powerful and empowering. Printed hand-outs can provide useful adjuncts to sessions and provide a written record of key issues for future reference. Similarly, pies charts can provide an objective way of identifying, quantifying, and challenging assumptions about inflated responsibility or the likelihood of events occurring.

The Internet provides a rich source of material to highlight key concepts such as cognitive biases or guided mindfulness exercises. Video clips form YouTube can be very powerful and provide a way of bringing the experience of another young person into the session to highlight a particular issue or skill. The materials need to be matched to the interests and developmental level of the young person to ensure that they are understandable and helpful and not perceived as patronising.

Technology

Adolescents are highly familiar with, and competent in, using computers, the Internet, and smart-phones. Technologies such as these are very appealing and offer a way of engaging with this age group (Boydell et al. 2014).

Laptop computers and smartphones may offer a more engaging way of completing diaries. The transportability of these devices can help the quick and accurate recording of mood, thoughts, or positive events as they occur. They can provide a way for young people to 'download their heads' when they notice any 'hot thoughts' or strong emotional reactions. Because young people are often texting and interacting with mobile devices briefly recording information such as this will not attract peer attention.

Smartphone cameras provide the young person with a way of recording difficult or challenging situations. Images can be reviewed to check some of the young person's thoughts or assumptions about what is happening and can help plan how to cope with difficult situations. The young person's photo-library can include pictures of their calming place which can remind and help them to create their image when required. Similarly, the young person can load positive coping statements or reminders about processes such as thought challenging (e.g. 4Cs see page 121) on to their home page to prompt them to challenge their thoughts.

The Internet provides a helpful way of researching and normalising common problems such as feeling anxious or low in mood. Celebrities who have suffered such conditions can be found and ways in which these celebrities learned to succeed identified as possible options for the young person to consider. Web sites which provide guidance and instructions on techniques such as mindfulness or relaxation can be accessed to facilitate and guide practice. Similarly, there is a wealth of useful videos of young people talking about their personal experiences of psychological problems and strategies they found helpful. Learning from other young people can be very powerful with video-stories and YouTube clips providing helpful ways to do this.

> CBT needs to be flexible and to be matched to the cognitive, linguistic, and perspective-taking abilities of the young person.

▶ Common problems when undertaking CBT with young people

Limited verbal skills

The process of CBT with young people may be less didactic than that with adults. Young people may adopt a more passive listening role during sessions. Whilst this may require greater input from the clinician, it does not necessarily imply that the young person is unable to engage in CBT. As previously highlighted, the clinician needs to be flexible in their approach and to adjust the materials to match the young person's preferences. In these situations, a greater use of non-verbal materials may be helpful with whiteboards and flip charts providing a useful way to communicate. Increasingly, the Internet is familiar and engaging for many young people and provides a way of bringing different experiences and perspectives in to the session. Video clips of young people talking about their experience of CBT and skills they found helpful are readily available for use. Similarly, there are many engaging videos and guided practice sessions available to learn skills such as mindfulness.

The clinician may also find it helpful to develop a more rhetorical approach with unforthcoming young people. This might, for example, involve guessing what the young person might reply to questions. Similarly, if the young person is reluctant to talk about themselves, then discussing a similar problem from the perspective of a third party maybe easier and result in more engagement. Finally, it may be useful to change the setting, so rather than sitting in the clinic, try going for a coffee or a walk and see if the young person becomes more communicative.

Limited cognitive skills

Whilst a basic level of cognitive skills is required to engage in CBT, the process can be adapted to meet the developmental needs of young people with limited abilities.

Presenting information more visually, using simpler language, and presenting abstract concepts in more concrete ways can make it easier for people with learning disabilities to engage in CBT (Whitaker 2001).

Memory problems can be overcome by the use of visual cues and prompts. A young person could learn to use traffic light system as a way of problem-solving (red: stop and think: amber: plan; green: try it out). They can be prompted to use this process at college or work by wrapping coloured strips around their pen. Similarly, tasks can be simplified with fewer decision points so that a young person could be helped to 'bail out' (i.e. walk away) of situations when they might lose their temper rather than learning a more complex set of problem-solving responses.

Similarly, cognitive tasks can be simplified through, for example, the use of self-instructional techniques (Meichenbaum 1975). This involves developing helpful self-statements such as 'I can . . .' which encourage the young person to cope whilst countering any negative or unhelpful automatic thoughts. Furthermore, as summarised in Chapter 1, 'Cognitive behaviour therapy:

theoretical origins, rationale, and techniques', CBT has developed over time with many interventions including behavioural methods. If cognitive skills are limited the cognitive demands can be matched to the young person's capacity whilst focusing more upon behavioural techniques.

Lack of engagement

Young people do not usually refer themselves for help and may not perceive any particular problems that they would like to change. If the young person is unable to identify any goals or changes they would like to make, then the use of CBT should be questioned. However, this requires careful exploration since the young person's inability to identify possible goals may be a result of their experience, i.e. 'this is the way it has always been and always will be'. Helping the young person to explore alternative, realistic possibilities may help them recognise that their situation could be different. Similarly a lack of motivation, as found, for example, with depressed young people, may result in the expression of reluctance and hopelessness. In these instances, motivational interviewing maybe helpful in securing the young person's commitment (Miller and Rollnick 1991). Motivational interviewing utilises basic counselling techniques such as empathy, positive regard, active listening, and cognitive-behavioural interventions such as positive restructuring to increase a person's commitment to change. However, if after a short period, the young person continues to be ambivalent, then this may not be the right time to pursue a CBT programme.

No responsibility for securing change

Young people may identify the difficulties and targets for change, but may not view themselves as responsible for achieving them. On occasions, this will be appropriate, but at other times, difficulties may be attributed to organic factors, e.g. 'this is me, I was born like this' or external factors that are not seen as within the individual's ability to change. A young person, for example, who is regularly in trouble at college or work may, attribute this externally as being unfairly picked e.g. 'if they didn't pick on me, then I wouldn't be in trouble'. Whether this is really the case, or a reflection of distorted or biased views needs to be assessed. However, the young person needs to be encouraged to suspend their views and to be prepared to at least explore their personal contribution to these events in order engage in CBT.

Difficulty accessing thoughts

If directly asked, 'What were you thinking', young people may be unable to identify and vocalise their thoughts. Careful listening will, however, reveal that beliefs, assumptions, and appraisals are often evident as they talk. At these times, it is often useful for the clinician to adopt the role described by Turk (1998) of the 'thought catcher', identifying important cognitions when they occur and bringing them to the attention of the young person. The clinician may stop the dialogue and bring the young person's attention to the cognitions they have just verbalised or alternatively, they may be held and summarised at a suitable time. For example, the clinician may listen to a young person's description of a recent 'hot' situation and then summarise the key feelings and associated thoughts that they identified.

Young people often confuse thoughts and feelings leading Belsher and Wilkes (1993) to highlight the need to 'chase the effect'. The authors suggest that particular attention be paid during clinical sessions to changes in emotion which are feedback to the young person in order to identify the associated cognitions, e.g. 'you seem to be thinking about something that is making you angry'. Often young people will require further help to discover their cognitions, and the clinician can either pursue Socratic questioning or provide a list of possible suggestions which the young person can reject or agree with. By a process of observation and careful questioning, the young person can be helped to become aware of the cognitions underlying their emotions.

Failure to undertake home assignments

CBT is an active process typically involving the gathering of information and the practice of skills outside of clinical sessions. Whilst some young people are interested and willing to undertake home-based assignments, others are unwilling and repeatedly fail to return with any material. This needs to be openly discussed with the young person, the importance of the assignments explained, and the extent of what can realistically be undertaken, if anything, agreed. Identifying an appropriate way of undertaking the task is also important. Young people may, for example, be reluctant to write a thought diary, but may be more interested in keeping a record on their computer or phone. Similarly, other young people maybe more motivated to e-mail their thoughts, whilst others may prefer to 'download their head' into a voice recorder.

Completing home-based assignments is not a pre-requisite during the self-awareness stage of CBT. The experiences, thoughts, and feelings of those who are unable to keep records can still be assessed during clinical sessions. They can be asked to talk through a recent difficult situation and the clinician can probe and explore the thoughts and feelings that accompanied the event.

However, home-based assignments are important during the skill development and consolidation phase. This is where the young person practices skills under everyday conditions to discover those that are helpful. Without practice, the young person will not be able to develop their new skills and learn to behave in different ways. By this stage, it is anticipated that the therapeutic relationship is open and strong enough to have this discussion and to see how home assignments can be made easier for the young person to undertake.

Focus shifting

Young people often have a short-term perspective and focus on the here and now. It is therefore not unusual when working with young people to find that major issues that formed the focus of a previous session miraculously disappear and are no longer problems. This focus shift can be disconcerting for clinicians and can result in problem-chasing rather than the systematic development of a comprehensive set of skills.

The resolution of a previous problem provides a useful opportunity for celebration and to develop the young person's self-efficacy. The young person can be helped to reflect and to explore what they did and how these ideas can be applied to other parts of their life that they find challenging. The clinician can relate this to the CBT model and can draw out important relationships between thinking and behaviour and highlight important coping strategies. Thus whilst the specific problem focus might shift, the underpinning CBT framework remains to provide the framework for reflection.

Working with egocentricity

During CBT, the young person needs to be non-judgemental and open to new ideas and explanations. This can be difficult for some young people who present in a very egocentric way and are convinced that their understanding is the only option. It is not uncommon to find that such a stance often results in the clinician attempting to persuade the young person that there are alternative explanations. However, this is often counter-productive and results in the young person defending their views more vigorously and becoming less willing to engage in any objective evaluation. Instead, it is useful to adopt an open and curious position in which the young person is helped to question their views through a Socratic dialogue. This process requires the clinician to adopt a reflective position in which the young person's views are acknowledged but not directly challenged. Instead, in a curious way, the clinician asks the young person to reflect upon new, inconsistent or contradictory information. The young person is encouraged to demonstrate how this information fits with their beliefs and assumptions or to consider how their views may need modification. Through this process, the young person is helped to critically appraise their views.

Significant family dysfunction

The dynamics within families are complex. This can result in young people being scapegoated and inappropriately being perceived as responsible for all the families' difficulties. In such situations, working with the young person on their own without addressing the wider family issues would not be appropriate.

Similarly, if a young persons' unhelpful cognitions are related to limited parental capabilities or concerning parental behaviour, then individual CBT would be inappropriate and unlikely to be effective (Kaplan, Thompson, and Searson 1995). The clinician needs to undertake a thorough assessment of comments such as 'my parents are always putting me down' to determine whether this is a cognitive distortion or an indication of significant family dysfunction. Determining this will indicate whether individual CBT or a more systemic approach is indicated.

'I get it, but I don't believe it'

There will be times when young people understand the aims and methods of CBT but appear to go through the process in an academic and detached way. Thoughts might be systematically challenged and alternatives developed, but the young person simply does not believe what they have discovered. Similarly, they might understand the aim of accepting and non-judgementally observing thoughts but are unable to stop arguing and engaging with them. Whilst there may be a need for further explanation and practice, it may become apparent that this approach does not work with this young person.

In the true spirit of partnership, this needs to be acknowledged and openly discussed. Whilst a guiding principle of CBT is for the young person to discover what works for them, it is equally important to discover what does not help. Potential barriers need to be explored, and the option of changing from a thought-challenging approach to one of observing and accepting (or vice versa) discussed. If the alternative is still not acceptable to the young person, then an alternative non-CBT approach should be considered.

Common problems in undertaking CBT with young people include the following:

Limited verbal or cognitive skills and difficulty accessing thoughts

Lack of engagement and/or problem ownership

Significant family dysfunction

Failure to undertake home-based assignments

Focus shifting

Problems understanding the approach

CHAPTER THREE

Thinking good, feeling better: overview of materials

Thinking Good, Feeling Better is a collection of materials that have adapted the concepts and strategies of cognitive behaviour therapy (CBT) for use with young people. The materials include methods and ideas from the traditional behaviour therapies and the second wave cognitive therapies in which young people are helped to develop skills to understand and actively change their behaviour and ways of thinking. *Thinking Good, Feeling Better* also draws on the 'third' wave models of CBT which focus on changing the nature of the relationship we have with our thoughts. These draw on ideas from mindfulness and acceptance and commitment therapy which promote non-judgemental compassionate awareness and acceptance.

Thinking Good, Feeling Better can be used flexibly and tailored towards the needs of the young person, their preferences, and the nature of their difficulties. The materials are not intended to be systematically delivered as a comprehensive programme. They do not provide, for example, a structured CBT or mindfulness intervention but instead draw on some of the ideas and techniques used in these models. Similarly, the materials are not focused upon a specific mental health problem such as depression or panic. They can be used with young people with a range of problems including anxiety, low mood, and anger. Finally, *Thinking Good, Feeling Better* can be used with young people with psychological problems as well as those who do not have any current problems. The materials will help to reduce psychological distress as well as developing skills to maintain and enhance psychological well-being.

A visual overview of the materials included in *Thinking Good, Feeling Better* is provided in Figure 3.1.

At the centre of the diagram is the traditional CBT materials focusing upon the core domains of the CBT model, what you think, how you feel, and what you do. Leading into this is a module about preparing for change which provides basic information about the CBT model and the goals and outcomes the young person would like to achieve. The final part of the model focuses upon how to keep well and summarises those skills that were particularly useful for the young person and what to do if problems re-emerge.

The outside circle draws on ideas from the new wave of CBT therapies. The skills are conceptualised as healthy habits designed to develop a new approach to life based on compassion, curiosity, mindful self-awareness, and acceptance. Instead of directly challenging and changing unhelpful cognitions, healthy habits focus on changing the nature of our relationship with our thoughts, feelings, and experiences. Healthy habits include mindfulness to promote self-awareness, acceptance, and tolerance of the events that occur, valuing who you are and what you do and a focus on kindness and personal strengths. These skills inform a keeping well plan to maintain positive well-being.

The distinction in Figure 3.1 between traditional CBT and the third wave models is primarily designed to highlight the different focus of these approaches. They are all concerned with reducing psychological distress, but traditional CBT achieves this by actively challenging and changing unhelpful thoughts, whilst the third wave methods primarily encourage observation and acceptance. Third wave CBT approaches are therefore conceptualised as healthy habits which form the basis of a

Thinking Good, Feeling Better: A Cognitive Behavioural Therapy Workbook for Adolescents and Young Adults, First Edition. Paul Stallard.
© 2019 John Wiley & Sons Ltd. Published 2019 by John Wiley & Sons Ltd.
Companion website: www.wiley.com/go/thinkinggood

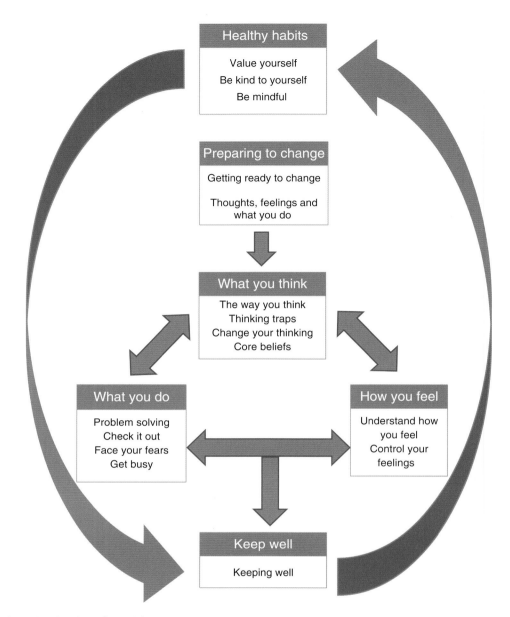

Figure 3.1 Overview of materials.

new approach to everyday life. However, it should be noted that these third wave models are very effective interventions in their own right. They are informed by research, have a clear theoretical underpinning which guides an extensive and comprehensive therapeutic intervention. The distinction is also arbitrary since there is overlap in some of the techniques used in traditional behaviour therapy, cognitive therapy, and the third wave approaches.

The materials and accompanying exercises in *Thinking Good, Feeling Better* cover the following topics:

1 Value yourself – recognise your strengths and take care of yourself

2 Be kind to yourself – accepting yourself for who you are

3 Be mindful – become a curious, non-judgemental observer

4 Getting ready to change – what would you like to be different?

5 Thoughts, feelings, and what you do – understanding the CBT model

6 The way you think – identifying helpful and unhelpful ways of thinking

7 Thinking traps – understanding common cognitive biases

8 Change your thinking – testing and developing more balanced and helpful ways of thinking

9 Core beliefs – discover your strong ways of thinking

10 Understand how you feel – recognise different emotions

11 Control your feelings – learn ways to manage your emotions

12 Problem-solving – learn how to tackle and overcome problems

13 Check it out – undertake experiments to test your thinking

14 Face your fears – break challenges into small steps

15 Get Busy – become active to improve your mood

16 Keeping well – remember the ideas that are most helpful for you

Each topic has an explanatory overview and some examples which relate the materials to issues and problems that the young person may find familiar. A series of worksheets accompany each topic and are designed to help the young person apply the information to their own particular difficulties. The worksheets can be flexibly used to focus on those issues or exercises that are most relevant for the young person. Worksheets can be downloaded and printed from the book's website.

▶ Value yourself

Summary

This introduces the concept of *self-esteem*, i.e. the way we see ourselves and what we do. The effect of high and low self-esteem on how we feel and behave is highlighted and how high self-esteem can be developed by recognising and focusing upon our *personal strengths* and achievements and the *positive things* that happen. Finally, young people are encouraged to *look after themselves* and to make sure that they eat and sleep well and keep physically active.

> ▪ Recognise your strengths
> ▪ Notice positive things
> ▪ Take care of yourself

Worksheets

Find your strengths encourages the young person to look at different aspects of themselves and their life in order to find their own strengths and achievements. A *positive diary* is included to help re-focus attention towards the positive things that happen. This is designed to counter the tendency to overlook or downplay positives by actively finding and recording achievements, successes, and those events that create positive emotions. *Celebrity self-esteem* asks young people to identify celebrities with high and low self-esteem and to describe how they behave and what they do. This can help to highlight some of the negative effects of low self-esteem and some of the skills and qualities that can contribute to high self-esteem. Finally, a *sleep diary* and *physical activity diary* are included for those young people who are worried about their sleep or are unsure whether they are active enough.

▶ Be kind to yourself

Summary

This section draws on ideas from compassion-focused therapy and acceptance and commitment therapy and encourages the young person to accept themselves for who they are rather than constantly criticising and finding fault with themselves and what they do. They are introduced to the idea of developing eight helpful habits. They are encouraged to treat themselves *like they would treat a friend* and to develop a kinder, less-critical inner voice. Instead of *kicking themselves when they are down*, they are encouraged to look after themselves when they are having a hard time. This includes learning to *forgive their mistakes* and to accept that these will happen and to notice and *celebrate what they achieve* rather than beating themselves up for the things they have not done. Instead of trying to be somebody different, they are encouraged to *accept who they are* and to *speak kindly to themselves*. Finally, they are encouraged to look for good things and to *find the good in others* and to *be kind to other people*.

> ■ Be kind to yourself
> ■ Forgive your mistakes
> ■ Accept who you are
> ■ Find the good in you and others

Worksheets

We are often more forgiving and supportive of our friends, but we treat ourselves in a harsh and critical way. *Treat yourself like a friend* helps the young person to look at the way they speak to themselves and asks them to compare this with how they would talk with a friend. *Look after yourself* is designed to counter the tendency to give ourselves a hard time when things go wrong. Instead of beating ourselves up, the young person is encouraged to do things to help themselves feel better. This theme is continued with *a kinder inner voice* where the young person is encouraged to develop and practice using kinder, less-critical self-statements. The final worksheet, *finding kindness*, encourages the young person to view the world differently and to actively seek out the kind things that happen.

▶ Be mindful

Summary

This section focuses on *mindfulness*, and the young person is introduced to the five steps of FOCUS. This involves the young person *focusing their attention* (F) and *observing* (O) *what is happening here and now in a curious way* (C). They are encouraged to *use their senses* (U) to maximise the experience. Finally, the young person is encouraged to *suspend judgement* (S) and to accept their thoughts and not to try to stop, change, or, engage with them. A number of ways in which mindfulness can be fitted into everyday life are described. The young person is encouraged to try mindful *breathing and eating* and to focus their attention and senses on *everyday activities* or objects we take for granted like walking or observing their pen. Finally, they are encouraged to *suspend judgement* and to try mindful *thinking*, where they stand back and observe their thoughts and feelings:

> ■ Focus attention on what is happening
> ■ Observe what is happening
> ■ Curious approach
> ■ Use your senses
> ■ Suspend judgement

Worksheets

Instructions are provided to help the young person integrate mindfulness into their everyday life. *Mindful breathing* is a quick exercise that can be done anywhere that helps the young person to focus on their breathing. *Mindful thinking* is a useful exercise when minds become cluttered with worries. The young person is encouraged to stand back and observe in a curious way the thoughts tumbling through their heads. *Mindful observation* helps the young person to fully focus their attention on everyday objects or places that are often taken for granted. Finally, *Do I really notice what I use* is a way of highlighting how little attention we pay to many of the familiar everyday objects we use.

▶ Getting ready to change

Summary

This section provides an introduction to CBT and the three major parts of the model: *what you think, how you feel, and what you do*. It highlights how unhelpful ways of thinking create unpleasant feelings which increase the chance that we will avoid, give up trying, or stop doing things. The worse we feel, the less we do, and the more time we have to think. We end up caught in a *negative trap* where our negative thoughts magically seem to come true.

The second part of this section checks whether the young person is *ready to try* to do things differently. This raises the question of whether they are ready to change and the need to suspend judgement and to be open to doing things differently. Identifying the *goals* the young person would like to achieve is important in ensuring that they are working towards an agreed outcome. The need for *SMART goals* – specific, meaningful, achievable, rewarding, and timely – is highlighted so that goals are clear. The *miracle question*, used in solution-focused therapy, is used to help the young person focus on the future and to think about how things would be different if they woke up and no longer had any problems.

> ▪ Introduction to the core elements of CBT, thoughts, feelings, and behaviour
> ▪ Identify personal goals

Worksheets

Are you ready to change is a way of assessing hopefulness, and whether this is the right time for the young person to engage in a process of change. If they are unsure whether things will change or if they can overcome their problems, it might be better to wait. *Cognitive behaviour therapy* is a very short explanatory hand-out that can be given to young people explaining CBT. *The miracle question* is drawn from solution-focused therapy and asks the young person to describe how the future will be different if they no longer had any problems. If the young person is having difficulty thinking about their goals, the miracle question can help to define them. Finally, *my goals* provide a week-by-week way of monitoring change, and the progress the young person is making to achieve their goals. The young person defines up to three goals and then rates the degree to which they are achieving them at the start of each session.

▶ Thoughts, feelings, and what you do

Summary

Further elaboration of CBT and the *negative trap* is provided with an explanation of different types of cognitions i.e. *core beliefs, assumptions,* and *automatic thoughts*. The ways in which core beliefs are activated and influence our assumptions and create the most accessible level of cognitions, *automatic thoughts*, is highlighted, and the effects of positive and negative thoughts upon *how you feel* and *what you do* is described. The *negative trap*, where negative thoughts produce unpleasant feelings that limit or restrict what you do is identified and the way this strengthens our original belief highlighted.

> ■ Introduction to core beliefs, assumptions, and automatic thoughts
> ■ Understanding the negative trap

Worksheets

The negative trap is a diagram that puts together the key parts of the cognitive model. This can be used as a hand-out to educate the young person into the cognitive model thereby providing a framework that joins together other sections of *Thinking Good, Feeling Better*.

Unhelpful thoughts is a worksheet that can help the young person become aware of the impact of their thoughts on how they feel and what they do. The young person is encouraged to write down a situation they find difficult and to try and capture some of the thoughts that tumble around in their head, the feelings they notice and how they behave.

▶ The way you think

Summary

The idea of *hot thoughts* is introduced to highlight how some ways of thinking create strong emotional reactions. Hot thoughts might be related to the cognitive triad, i.e. how we see ourselves, how we expect to be treated, or about the future. *Automatic thoughts* can be *helpful*, make us feel good, and encourage us to face challenges and focus on our strengths, successes, and achievements. They can also be *unhelpful*, make us feel unpleasant, and stop us from doing things by being negative, critical, and biased. The way we listen and accept our thoughts as true without stopping to question or challenge them is emphasised and the way this perpetuates the negative trap highlighted.

> ■ Helpful thoughts are motivating and produce pleasant emotions
> ■ Unhelpful thoughts are demotivating and produce unpleasant emotions

Worksheets

Three worksheets are provided to help young people become more aware of their thoughts. *Check your thoughts* asks the young person to keep a list of the thoughts that race through their mind when they notice a change in how they are feeling. They are asked to look for thoughts relating to the cognitive triad, i.e. about themselves, how they will be treated, and/or what they think will happen. *Hot thoughts* is a structured diary where the young person is asked to record the day and time, what they were doing, what was the strong emotion, and what thoughts were racing through their mind. Some young people might prefer to make their own diary on their computer or to email their hot thoughts. On other occasions, young people may struggle to identify their thoughts so instead of trying to find them, they are encouraged to simply *download your head*. This can be done by writing down whatever they notice tumbling through their heads. The young person needs to know that they may be embarrassed by what they write down or be unable to make sense of what they are thinking. This is fine, the task is to try to catch any thoughts that are tumbling around in their head and causing distress.

▶ Thinking traps

Summary

Cognitive distortions and biases are introduced as *thinking traps* where we learn to think in unhelpful and biased ways. There are five main types of thinking traps with 11 common cognitive distortions being highlighted. The negative filter is the first thinking trap, where anything positive is filtered out and goes unrecognised. This happens in two ways: '*Negative Glasses*' (i.e. selective abstraction) is where the young person is biased towards the negative things that happen, and '*Positive doesn't count*' (disqualifying the positive) where anything positive is dismissed as unimportant or irrelevant. The second trap is blowing things up where negative events become more important than they really are. This happens in three main ways: '*Magnifying the negative*' (magnification) is where inflated importance is attached to any small negative things that happen, whilst '*Disaster thinking*' (catastrophisation) is where the young person ends up thinking the worse possible outcome. Finally, '*All-or-nothing thinking*' (binary thinking) is where we think in extreme ways, and there is nothing in between. The third thinking trap is predicting failure (arbitrary inferences) where we make predictions and often assume the worse. The two common traps are the '*Mind Reader*' who assumes that they know what others are thinking and the '*Fortune Teller*' who knows what will happen. The fourth type of thinking trap is where we are down on ourselves which can happen in two main ways. '*Dustbin labels*' (labelling) is where we assign ourselves a general negative label which we apply to all parts of our life. The second is '*Blame me*' (personalisation) where we assume responsibility for any negative things that happen. The final trap is where we set ourselves up to fail (unrealistic expectations) which can happen in two ways. '*Should and must*' are where we set unrealistically high expectations about how we and others should behave. '*Expecting to be perfect*' is where we set ourselves unachievable standards which we constantly fail to achieve thereby strengthening our beliefs that we are a failure.

- Identification of common thinking traps
- Thought monitoring and identification of personal traps

Worksheets

Thinking traps is a hand-out for young people summarising the main thinking traps and asking them to note down any examples they might notice. *Thoughts and feelings* is a structured diary which builds on the earlier hot thoughts diary by asking the young person to both record their thoughts and whether they have fallen into a thinking trap, if so which one.

▶ Change your thinking

Summary

Once the young person is able to identify their thoughts and common thinking traps, the next stage is *thought checking* where thoughts are systematically checked and tested. The young person is introduced to a four-step process in which they are encouraged to '*Catch*' their unhelpful ways of thinking and to '*Check*' whether they are making things out to be worse than they really are. The third step requires them to '*Challenge*' their thoughts by actively searching for any contradictory evidence they might have overlooked, forgotten, or dismissed as unimportant. This leads to the final step where the young person is encouraged to reflect on what they have discovered to '*Change*' their way of thinking to something that is more balanced and helpful and better fits the evidence.

It can be hard for young people to challenge their own negative ways of thinking. On these occasions, it may be easier to challenge these thoughts by taking another perspective and asking *what someone else would say*. Ask the young person what their best friend or someone they respect would say if they heard them thinking like this. Alternatively, what they would say to their best friend if they had these thoughts.

Finally, *dealing with worries* discusses ways to deal with constant worries. Worries are classified as those we can do something about and the 'what if' worries we have no control over. The need to limit worry is emphasised by establishing a worry time, devoted to worrying. Worries that occur throughout the day are noted, but worrying is delayed until worry time. During worry time, the worries are sorted, and solutions found for those we can do something about. We are encouraged to accept and let go those worries we can do nothing about.

> ▪ Cognitive evaluation
> ▪ Cognitive restructuring
> ▪ Third-party perspective
> ▪ Limit time spent worrying

Worksheets

Thought checking guides the young person through the four-step process of challenging their thoughts. Writing this down on paper can be a powerful way of helping to discover thinking traps and overlooked information. *What would someone else say* helps the young person to identify their thoughts and to consider and challenge these from the perspective of a friend or another person they respect. *Dealing with worries* provides a worry diary and helps the young person to sort these into those they can do something about and those they need to accept.

▶ Core beliefs

Summary

Sometimes it is hard to change the way we think because our ways of thinking are so strong, rigid, and powerful. These are our *core beliefs* which can be identified by repeatedly asking the question '*So what does it mean?*' The process involves taking a commonly heard thought and repeatedly asking the question '*So what does it mean?*' until the core belief emerges. Because core beliefs are very powerful and resistant to any challenge, the aim is to find evidence that helps to put limits around them. This can be achieved by actively collecting evidence that the belief is *not always true*. If this is still difficult, then it might be helpful to *talk with someone* else.

> ▪ Identification of core beliefs
> ▪ Challenging and testing core beliefs

Worksheets

So what does it mean is the downward arrow exercise that helps to discover core beliefs (Burns 1980). After identifying a common or powerful thought, the young person is asked, 'So what (if this were true) does this mean' until the core belief is identified.

Once identified, *is it always true* can be used to record any evidence that this belief may not always be 100% true. This can help the young person to put some limits around powerful ways of thinking such as 'I am a failure' to something like 'I might fail at my academic lessons, but I am successful at drama'.

Finally, *my beliefs* are the Schema Questionnaire for Children (Stallard and Rayner 2005; Stallard 2007) and provide a way of assessing how strongly the child identifies with a set of 15 common beliefs. This provides the clinician with an insight into the young person's beliefs that can be used to discover why the same difficulties keep re-occurring or why they end up in the same negative traps.

▷ Understand how you feel

Summary

This section focuses upon affective education and aims to increase awareness of different feelings by helping the young person to understand their *body signals*. The common unpleasant emotions of *stress, depression,* and *anger* are discussed, and the relationship between feelings, thoughts, and behaviour is highlighted.

> ■ Affective education
> ■ Affective monitoring

Worksheets

Worksheets are included to raise awareness of common body signals for *feeling down, feeling anxious,* and *feeling angry*. These can be completed individually or in a group. Completing in a group allows young people to discover some of the more common emotional signals and how some signals might be shared by different emotions (e.g. feel hot and red in the face). This can help to gain a better understanding of how others might be feeling whilst helping them to develop their own emotional literacy so that they can intervene earlier to manage their feelings.

Often young people are unaware of how common anxiety and depression are. *Do others feel like me* encourages young people to use the Internet to find out about this and to identify famous celebrities who have suffered and how they overcame their problems. The *feeling diary* is a way of helping young people discover that feelings don't randomly happen, but that they are triggered by specific situations or thoughts. *Mood monitoring* shows how feelings change throughout the day and helps to identify those times which are particularly difficult.

▷ Control your feelings

Summary

This section focuses on the development of emotional management skills and provides a number of different strategies that can be used in different situations. Some methods will inevitably be more helpful than others, fit better with ideas that the young person already uses, or can more readily be integrated into their everyday life. The idea is to develop a toolbox of methods that can be used in different situations.

Different ways of undertaking progressive muscle relaxation exercises are explained. *Relaxation exercises* describe exercises to tense and relax each major muscle group whilst *quick relaxation* tenses muscle groups together. *Physical activity* uses everyday activities that are already enjoyed as a way of tensing and relaxing muscles. A method of controlled breathing, *4-5-6 breathing* can be used as a quick way of regaining emotional control and calming down. *Mind games* are distraction exercises where attention is focused away from unhelpful thoughts or body signals towards neutral, external stimuli. These can provide short-term relief or help to face a challenge but are not long-term strategies that should be encouraged. *Change the feeling* encourages the young person to actively do something to change how they are feeling. If feeling sad, engage in an activity that creates the opposite reaction and makes the young person happy or laugh, or if feeling angry, find an activity that makes them feel calm. *Soothe yourself* is an idea used in Dialectical Behaviour Therapy in which the major senses are stimulated to soothe and calm the young person. Finally, the young person is encouraged to *talk to someone* and to draw up a list of contacts that they can talk with about how they are feeling or who make them feel better.

- Relaxation
- Physical activity
- Calming imagery
- Controlled breathing
- Distraction
- Self-soothing
- Talk with someone

Worksheets

Relaxing diary is a summary of how the young person felt before and after completing relaxation exercises. They are encouraged to rate the strength of their anxiety before and after relaxation. This can help to highlight potential changes in anxiety and focus on any problems where relaxation did not seem to be helpful. *Activities that help you feel better* records sporting activities, physical activities, or other physical things that the young person undertakes or enjoys. This provides a menu of physical activities that the young person could try to use when they feel stressed, angry, or unhappy. The idea of calming imagery is introduced in *my calming place* which helps the young person to create a multi-sensory image of a real or imaginary place that they find relaxing. When they become stressed, the young person can escape to their calming place to regain control and relax.

Change the feeling asks the young person to list the things they do which make them feel relaxed, happy, and calm. The list provides a menu of activities they can use to help them feel better. *Soothing toolbox* encourages the young person to think about the things they find pleasant and which stimulate each of their senses. These could be pleasurable smells (e.g. scented candle and coffee), tactile sensations (e.g. feel of a soft toy and warm bath), tastes (e.g. chocolate and mint), sights (e.g. photos and clouds in the sky) or sounds (e.g. music and birds singing). Once identified, these can be collated and put together in a soothing toolbox for use when required. *Talk to someone* encourages the young person to pull together a list of people they could contact and talk with about how they are feeling or who make them feel better. This helps the young person to think about what they want to tell someone, what they want them to do, and how and when they will contact them.

▶ Problem-solving

Summary

Every day we need to make a number of decisions. Some decisions are straightforward, but others are more complicated, and there may not be one simple answer. The consequences of our decisions can create problems. We may put decisions off or rush in without fully thinking things through. We may become emotional with our feelings clouding our judgement or are very fixed and rigid in our ideas and unable to see any other options.

A six-step approach to *problem-solving* is introduced which encourages the young person to consider a range of options and to appraise the short- and long-term consequences for themselves and the others involved. Once assessed, the young person makes their decision and afterwards reflects on whether they would choose this option again.

Some problems and challenges feel very big and difficult to tackle. Rather than avoiding these, the young person is encouraged to *break it down* into smaller, more manageable steps. Each small step moves the young person closer to achieving their overall goal.

> - Problem-solving
> - Break challenges into small steps

Worksheets

A *problem-solving* worksheet is provided that can be used to guide the young person through the six-step process. *Break it down* can be used to identify some of the smaller steps that will lead the young person to their overall goal. When defining the steps, it is important that they are challenging but not too large. The aim is to increase confidence and motivation by successful completion of each smaller step.

▷ Check it out

Summary

The process of thought challenging can be a very effective way of helping young people to develop more balanced and helpful ways of thinking. There will however be times when the young person's thoughts are very strong, rigid, and resistant to this thought-checking process. At these times, *experiments* are very helpful ways of objectively testing beliefs and predictions. These are undertaken in a safe way and are designed to genuinely check out what happens rather than to prove or disprove a particular way of thinking.

Another way of objectively checking thoughts and beliefs is through *surveys and searches*. These are particularly useful ways of exploring alternative explanations for events and for checking the views of others. The Internet and social media provide a convenient and accessible way of gathering information. *Responsibility pies* are a useful way of helping to put limits around beliefs and assumptions and of visually acknowledging possible contributors to events.

> - Test predictions
> - Behavioural experiments, surveys and searches

Worksheets

The check-it-out worksheet provides a guide of the steps involved in designing and carrying out an experiment. The step in which the young person is encouraged to reflect on what they have found out is particularly important and compares their prediction with what actually occurred. *Surveys and searches* provides a template for undertaking a survey and again encourages the young person to reflect on what they have learned and how this new information can be integrated into their beliefs and assumptions. The *responsibility pie* is a useful way of getting things in perspective by listing all the possible reasons why something might have happened. Each reason is assigned a slice of the pie with the size of the slice reflecting how much each contributed to the outcome.

▶ Face your fears

Summary

This section is helpful for young people who are avoiding things that make them anxious. Whilst avoidance may result in short-term relief, it can severely limit what the young person is able to do and does not help them learn how to beat their worries and cope. The young person is encouraged to *face their fears* and reclaim their life by taking *small steps* to climb their *fear ladder*. Breaking their fear into smaller steps helps to make each step more manageable and will take the young person closer to achieving their overall goal. When facing their fear, it is important that the young person stays in the situation until their anxiety comes down. This helps the young person learn that their fears are not as bad as they imagined, that anxiety does come down, and most importantly, that they can cope.

- Hierarchy development
- Systematic desensitisation
- Exposure

Worksheets

Small steps provides a way of breaking down a large fear, e.g. of talking with people, into a number of specific situations. The fear of talking with people might result in the young person avoiding parties, sleeping over at friends, going into the canteen at lunchtime, travelling on the school bus, going into town, asking for help at school, or asking for things in a shop. The *fear ladder* invites the young person to select one of the small steps they have identified and to work out the smaller steps they need to undertake to achieve it. Each small step is rated for anxiety and is then placed up the ladder in order of difficulty. *Face your fears* is the final stage when the young person faces the first step on their fear ladder. This helps the young person to attend to their anxiety and to reflect on what they have learned and achieved. The need for self-reinforcement and to reward success should be emphasised and the young person should be encouraged to celebrate their achievements, no matter how small. The young person then takes the next step on their fear ladder as they learn to overcome their anxiety and reclaim their life.

▶ Get busy

Summary

This section is helpful for young people who feel low in their mood and have stopped doing things. As the young person does less, they have more thinking time to rehearse what has happened or to worry about what will happen. *What you do – how you feel* helps the young person discover the link between activity and how they feel and can help to identify those times of the day that are most difficult. Once identified, activity rescheduling can help to experiment and *change what you do*. This encourages the building in of more mood-lifting feel-good activities at those times associated with low mood. Finally, the idea of behavioural activation is introduced as *have more fun*. The young person is encouraged to gradually build in more enjoyable, social, active or activities that create a sense of achievement into their life. The initial goal is to become active not to feel better. The change in mood will probably come later.

- Activity monitoring
- Activity rescheduling
- Behavioural activation

What you do — how you feel is a psychoeducational activity diary exploring the link between mood and activity. The young person describes what they are doing throughout a day, how they felt, and how strong the feeling was. *Have more fun* helps the young person to think about the activities they find or have found enjoyable. This can be hard if they are feeling down and so the young person is encouraged to list the things they use to enjoy but have now stopped, what they like but don't do very often, and the things they want to do but haven't got round to doing. The young person can then select one or two of these activities to try. *Plan more fun* can help to structure this by encouraging the young person to decide when they will do and to record what happened.

▶ Keeping well

Summary

This section focuses on keeping well and relapse prevention. It highlights an eight-point keeping well plan which encourages the young person to identify *what helped* them in terms of important messages and skills they discovered. They are encouraged to *build them into their life* so that they continue to *practice* their helpful skills. They are prepared to *expect setbacks* and are encouraged to see these as short term. *Knowing your warning signs* and *watch out for difficult times* helps the young person to prevent future difficulties by watching out for signs that unhelpful habits are returning and to prepare for challenging situations or events. Finally, the young person is encouraged *to be kind* to themselves during a setback and to *stay positive*, remembering their strengths and what they have achieved.

- Relapse prevention
- Keeping well

Worksheets

The young person is encouraged to develop a *keeping well* plan in which they write down key messages, ideas, relaxation strategies, and cognitive skills they found helpful. *My warning signs* is designed to increase early detection of unhelpful ways of thinking and changes in emotions and behaviour that might suggest a setback. Finally, *difficult situations* can help the young person to prepare for future challenges. Identifying potentially difficult events or situations can help the young person to think through a coping plan and to practice the skills that will help them to be successful.

Value yourself

The way you think about yourself, your **self-esteem**, is important. Self-esteem is how much you respect and value yourself for who you are and for what you do. It affects how you feel and how you behave. Self-esteem can either be **low** or **high**.

People with **low** self-esteem:

▸ are **very self-critical** and beat themselves up

▸ are **not confident** and are unsure about trying new things

▸ often feel they are **not good enough**

▸ focus on their **weaknesses and failures**

▸ **overlook success**

▸ **feel worthless**

▸ are **reluctant to face challenges**

sarahdesign/Shutterstock

People with **low self-esteem** don't respect themselves or value what they do.

People with **high** self-esteem:

▸ **respect** themselves for who they are

▸ **are confident** and willing to try new things

▸ **value** what they do

▸ **recognise their strengths** and qualities

▸ **are proud** of their achievements

▸ **feel worthy** of being happy and of doing well

▸ are **prepared to face challenges**

Thinking Good, Feeling Better: A Cognitive Behavioural Therapy Workbook for Adolescents and Young Adults, First Edition. Paul Stallard.
© 2019 John Wiley & Sons Ltd. Published 2019 by John Wiley & Sons Ltd.
Companion website: www.wiley.com/go/thinkinggood

People with **high self-esteem** are more positive and value themselves.

How does self-esteem develop?

We are not born with high or low self-esteem. It develops over time and is shaped by important things that happen.

Your important relationships with family, teachers, and friends, and what they say about you, and how they treat you

▶ If you are always criticised or told off for getting things wrong, you may never feel good enough.

▶ If you have lots of friends, you may feel valued.

The expectations and standards that you and others set and your achievements and failures

▶ If you are always self-critical and never satisfied with what you do, you may not respect yourself.

▶ If you recognise your efforts and what you achieve, you may feel proud.

Important events and experiences as you grow up

▶ If you were bullied or were seriously ill, you may feel worthless or weak.

▶ If you are successful with your school work or at a sport, you may feel confident.

Can you change self-esteem?

Yes. You can probably think about many people who have been able to improve their self-esteem. It could be a family member, a friend, athlete, musician, or famous celebrity. There are many examples of people who had low self-esteem but were able to change it to become more confident and to value and respect themselves.

To improve self-esteem you need **to find your strengths**, to **celebrate the positive** things that happen, and to **value yourself** for who you are.

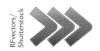

RFvectors/ Shutterstock

Find your strengths

People with low self-esteem are very self-critical and often focus on their weaknesses and the things that go wrong. They criticise and beat themselves up and end up feeling useless or worthless.

Try to find **your strengths**. Even though it may be hard, there will be times when you are able **to be successful**, **to cope**, to face, and **deal with challenges.**

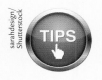

sarahdesign/ Shutterstock

To find your strengths, look for things that are **going well**, that **you enjoy**, and the challenges **you have coped** with. Try to find strengths and skills in **different areas.**

- ▶ **What do you do in your free time?** What are you good at or enjoy? Playing music, gaming, acting, art, or looking after animals?

- ▶ **What physical activity do you like?** Walking, dance, gym, football, cycling, or swimming?

- ▶ **What do you do at college or work?** What would your manager say about you? Do you try hard, complete assignments on time, and contribute to discussions.

- ▶ **What have you achieved?** Have you done anything special? Have you done well in a contest, been singled out for a special mention, or been selected for anything special.

- ▶ **What do people like about you?** Why do people want to be with you? Are you kind, caring, good fun, strong willed, have good ideas, or good at arranging things?

- ▶ **Your relationships?** What would you friends or family say about you? Are you a good listener, loyal friend, or willing to help?

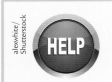

HELP You can't be good at everything, so you may not find strengths in every area. If you find it hard to find any strengths ask your friends, teachers, or parents.

Use your strengths

Once you have found your strengths, the next step is to think how you can use these to help you cope with future problems and challenges.

How did you develop your skills?

▸ You probably weren't very good at the start, so how did you learn to become so good?

▸ Did you practice, were you determined, did someone help you?

▸ Can you use these ideas to help you cope with your challenges?

How does physical activity make you feel?

▸ When you do physical activity, does it make you feel better?

▸ Does it give you a sense of achievement or pride?

▸ Can you do something physical when you are feeling down or stressed to make yourself feel better?

How do you cope with challenges?

▸ Are there things you do at college or work which can help with other problems?

▸ Do you research what to do, work with others, or write a plan?

▸ Can these ideas help you deal with challenges in other parts of your life?

How did you manage your achievements?

▸ How did you manage to stand out?

▸ How did you motivate yourself and feel confident to do this?

▸ Can you use this learning to cope with other challenges?

How can you use your qualities?

▸ Can your personal strengths help you with your problems?

▸ Are you strong minded, creative, or well organised?

▸ Can these skills help you overcome your problems?

How can your relationships help?

▷ Is there someone you trust or value who could help?

▷ What would they say about you social skills that are helpful?

▷ Can your social skills and friendships help you deal with challenges?

 TIPS Think about how you **gained your skills** and how you can **apply them** to those parts of your life that are not going so well

 ## Find and celebrate the positive

Once you have found your strengths you need to focus on the **positive** things that happen and to **celebrate** what you do. This will help you feel better, to be more confident, and to have a more balanced view about yourself. Look for

▷ the **good things** that happen

▷ the things **you enjoy**

▷ the times **you have coped**

▷ **what you achieve** no matter how small

 TIPS A useful way to do this is to keep a **positive diary**. Find at least one positive thing that has happened each day. Watching your list grow will help you remember that positive things do happen.

When you complete your diary try to find things that

▷ **made you feel good** – watched a funny film, listened to some music, or a long hot bath

▷ **you enjoyed** – talked with your friend, went for a walk, or baked a cake

▷ **you coped with** – joined in with a discussion went somewhere new, or talked with someone you don't know very well

▷ **you achieved** – finished an assignment, controlled your temper, or helped at home

When you feel down or hopeless look through your diary. This will help you to keep things in balance and remind you that although it can be tough **good things do happen** and **you can cope**.

Look after yourself

If you have low self-esteem, you may not value yourself. You may not think you are important and may not look after yourself as well as you could. You may not **eat** very well, have problems **sleeping**, drink too much **alcohol** or don't do much **physical activity**, and become unfit. By taking care of yourself, you may start to feel better.

Diet

A balanced diet and regular meals will **help your physical and mental health**. A healthy diet will help control your weight and will prevent some diseases linked with being overweight such as diabetes, heart problems, and high blood pressure.

There are lots of ways you can have a healthy diet. Sometimes there is too much advice, and it all feels overwhelming. If you want to keep it simple, try these **five tips**.

▷ **Eat breakfast**. Breakfast can help you to concentrate and can help you control your weight.

▷ **Eat regular meals**. If you skip meals you may find that you are constantly snacking on unhealthy foods which may increase your weight.

▷ **Eat as much fresh fruit or vegetables** as you can each day.

▷ **Limit sugary foods and drinks** as these can lead to weight gain and increase health problems.

▷ **Drink plenty of water** at least 1.5–2 litres of water per day to stop you becoming dehydrated.

Sleep

A good night's sleep is important for keeping you well and healthy. This is really important for young people who need more sleep than adults as their bodies and brains are growing.

There are two common sleep problems

▶ not enough sleep or

▶ problems falling asleep

How much sleep do I need?

How much sleep you need depends on you, but most people **need around seven to nine hours** each night. Everyone has bad nights and will wake up feeling tired. If this keeps happening, you may feel

▶ **constantly tired**

▶ fall **asleep during the day**

▶ have **problems concentrating**

▶ may **overeat**

▶ drink lots of **caffeine, sugary, or energy drinks**

▶ feel **irritable and angry**

▶ may feel **sad** and **frustrated**

If you wake up and feel refreshed, are able to concentrate, don't nap or fall asleep during the day, then you are probably having enough sleep.

If you wake up and feel tired, find it hard to get out of bed, can't concentrate, or nap or fall asleep during the day, you are probably not getting enough sleep.

You can check how much sleep you are getting by keeping a **sleep diary**. Check what time you go to bed, how long it takes to fall asleep, how many times you wake in the night, when you wake in the morning, and when you get up.

I'm not getting enough sleep

If you are not getting enough sleep, **try changing your internal clock**. This programmes us to wake up and fall asleep at certain times. You may notice that you wake up at the same time at the weekends as you do during the week. This is because your internal clock is set to wake you up and doesn't care what day it is.

If you are not getting enough sleep, then

- keep a **sleep diary** and check what time you are going to bed

- now bring your bed time forward and go to bed **half an hour earlier**

- make sure you **get up at the same time** in the morning and **don't nap** during the day

- if after a few days you are still feeling tired, bring your bedtime forward **another half an hour** until you feel that you are having enough sleep

 You can **re-set your internal clock** by going to bed half an hour earlier. If after a few days you are still feeling tired, go to bed another half hour earlier until you have enough sleep

I can't get off to sleep

Not being able to fall asleep is very frustrating. You may find that the harder, you try to sleep the more awake you become.

The most useful way to help yourself sleep well is to get a **good night-time routine**.

- **Make your bedroom a calm, quiet, sleep friendly place.** Make sure your bedroom is not too hot or cold and is as quiet and as comfortable as you can make it.

- **Have a wind-down** period before bed and do things that help you to relax – milky drink, bath/shower, watch TV, read a book, or listen to music.

- **Avoid activities that keep you wake** or might stimulate you like physical exercise and gaming.

- **Turn off light-emitting devices** such as computer screens, tables, and smart-phones at least one hour before bed. They produce blue light which affects the levels of the natural sleep-inducing hormone melatonin we produce.

▶ **Avoid drinks with caffeine** in the evening. Drinks like coffee, tea, and fizzy drinks contain caffeine which can stop you falling asleep.

▶ **Don't drink or eat too much** before you go to bed. You might feel uncomfortable and find it hard to sleep.

▶ **Decide on a set bedtime** and go to bed at that time each night.

▶ **Keep a sleep diary** to check how you are doing. Check what time you go to bed, how long it took to fall asleep, how many times you woke in the night, when you woke in the morning, and when you got up.

▶ **Cut down on alcohol**, cigarettes, and recreational drugs that keep you awake or disturb your sleep.

▶ **Try to exercise** each day so that you feel tired when you go to bed and ready to sleep.

If you are still awake after 20 minutes, then get out of bed. You want to train your body to sleep, not be awake, in your bed. Do something calming like reading a book, listening to music, or doing a puzzle book and then go back to bed and try again.

A **regular bedtime routine** will help you to wind down and prepare for sleep. Avoid screens and things that might stimulate you.

Alcohol

People often use alcohol to change how they feel and may feel calmer, happier, or less worried when they drink.

Alcohol can also work in different ways and may strengthen your unpleasant feelings so that you become more unhappy or aggressive.

If you are going to drink alcohol, then

▶ **Drink in moderation** – the safe drinking guidance recommends no more than 14 units each week.

▶ **Don't drink every day** – have three or four alcohol-free days each week.

▶ **Don't binge** – if you do, then make sure that someone is around to look after you and keep you safe.

It is not helpful to use alcohol to cope with your feelings. The effects will not last, and you will feel even worse after the alcohol wears off. Try to find other ways to manage your emotions.

Physical activity

Regular physical activity can help prevent serious health problems such as heart disease, high blood pressure, and diabetes and can reduce the risk of mental health problems like anxiety and depression.

Exercise can reduce feelings of stress and help you keep a healthy weight. The chemicals your brain releases when you exercise can make you feel good.

Try to do **moderate physical activity** which raises your heart and breathing rate for 30 minutes, five **times each week**. Find things you enjoy and which can be built into your routine.

Find some physical activities you enjoy:

▶ Training, running, jogging, swimming, gymnastics, or cycling

▶ Ball games such as football, netball, basketball, rugby, hockey, or cricket

▶ Everyday activities such as walking the dog, learning a dance routine, changing your bedroom around, skipping, and washing a car

▶ Get a dance or exercise DVD to use at home

Build activity into your daily routine:

▶ Get off the bus one stop earlier and walk

▶ Walk up the stairs instead of taking the escalator

▶ Cycle or walk to the shops instead of having a lift in a car

Exercise for 30 minutes each day, five times per week:

▶ If 30 minutes seems too much, start with 10 minutes each day and build up your activity each week

▶ If you can't do 30 minutes in one go, try two 15-minute periods each day

▶ If you don't feel like doing anything, then set yourself a more achievable goal and remember – any activity is better than none.

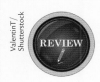

People with high self-esteem value and respect themselves, what they do, and what they achieve.

You can improve your self-esteem by noticing and using your strengths. Find the positive things that happen and look after yourself.

If you take care of yourself, you will feel better and be more able to cope with problems and challenges.

Find your strengths

Sometimes we forget or overlook our strengths and skills and focus on what we can't do. Remembering what you are good at can help you

▶ feel good about yourself

▶ feel more confident

▶ to face challenges and to tackle any problems

Find you strengths and write them in the boxes below.

What I do (e.g. music, art, acting, gaming, or looking after animals)

Activities I like (e.g. walking, jogging, dance, keep fit, or swim)

What I do at school (e.g. lessons you like, or things you are good at)

My achievements (e.g. learned something new or done something special)

Nice things about me (e.g. kind, try hard, clever, good listener, or funny)

Relationships – Friends/family (popular, trusted, kind, and helpful)

Positive diary

We are very good at noticing the negative things that happen but often overlook or rubbish the good things.

To become more balanced about what goes on in life write down, at least one positive thing that happens each day. This could be something

▶ you enjoyed

▶ you coped with

▶ you achieved

▶ made you feel good

Day	What happened

Watching the list grow will help you see that good things do happen.

Celebrity self-esteem

Self-esteem is the way we think about ourselves and what we do. People with high self-esteem

▶ respect and value themselves

▶ are confident

▶ recognise their strengths and are proud of their achievements

Think of a famous person, celebrity, film star, sports person, or musician you respect who has high self-esteem and another who has low self-esteem. How do they behave and what do they do?

> A celebrity with high self-esteem is:
>
>
> How they behave and what they do is:

> A celebrity with low self-esteem is:
>
>
> How they behave and what they do is:

How do you rate your self-esteem?

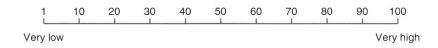

| 1 | 10 | 20 | 30 | 40 | 50 | 60 | 70 | 80 | 90 | 100 |

Very low   Very high

Sleep diary

If you don't think you are sleeping enough, try keeping this diary and see if there are any patterns.

	Example	Monday	Tuesday	Wednesday	Thursday	Friday	Saturday	Sunday
What did you do in the hour before you went to bed?	Played X box							
What time did you go to bed?	11.15							
What time did you fall asleep?	01.20							
How many times did you wake in the night?	None							
What time did you wake up?	09.30							
What time did you get out of bed?	11.00							
How was your sleep? 1 2 3 4 5 Very bad Very Good	4							

Make sure that you have a calming night-time routine and try to go to bed and get up at a similar time each day.

Physical activity diary

Complete this diary to check how much physical activity you do each week. Moderate physical activity will

▶ raise your heart rate

▶ increase your breathing

▶ make you feel warm

	Example	Monday	Tuesday	Wednesday	Thursday	Friday	Saturday	Sunday
What did you do and for how long?	Walked the dog 10 min							
	PE at school 30 min							
	Dance DVD 15 min							
Total moderate activity	55 min							

You should try to do 30 minutes of moderate physical activity for 5 days each week.

Be kind to yourself

We are not always very good at taking care of ourselves. We **are often very self-critical**. We beat ourselves up, criticise what we do, and blame ourselves for things that go wrong or feel ashamed if we are not perfect.

From an early age we are encouraged to be successful, to work hard, to be competitive, and to compare ourselves against others. This helps to motivate us, but can become a problem when we:

▶ are **never satisfied** with what we do or achieve

▶ **blame ourselves** for everything that goes wrong

▶ become **fixed on our imperfections and failures**

▶ never **acknowledge our strengths or celebrate our successes**

We develop a **critical inner voice**. We are unkind to ourselves. We are constantly criticising ourselves which makes us feel even worse.

Instead of tearing ourselves apart, we **need to accept that**

▶ things will **go wrong**

▶ we **are not perfect**

▶ we **will make mistakes**

▶ **unkind things do happen**

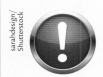

sarahdesign/
Shutterstock

> We need to **be kinder** to ourselves. We need to stop being so critical and start to feel comfortable with who we are, acknowledge our strengths, and to celebrate what we achieve.

Thinking Good, Feeling Better: A Cognitive Behavioural Therapy Workbook for Adolescents and Young Adults, First Edition. Paul Stallard.
© 2019 John Wiley & Sons Ltd. Published 2019 by John Wiley & Sons Ltd.
Companion website: www.wiley.com/go/thinkinggood

Eight helpful habits

Being kind to yourself will probably feel odd. You are used to listening to your inner critic, so changing this may take time. Try practicing these helpful habits to help you learn to be kinder to yourself.

Treat yourself like you would treat a friend

We are often quick to find our faults and to criticise ourselves. Our **critical inner voice** will tell us that we are *'useless'*, *'a failure'* or *'weak'* or call us names like *'stupid'*, *'idiot'* or *'looser'*. As we beat ourselves up we end up feeling even more stressed, angry, or down.

We are usually much harder on ourselves than we would be on someone else. What would you say to your friend if you heard them being very critical?

> ▶ If your friend put on some clothes and said, *'I look fat in these jeans'*. You probably wouldn't say, *'Yes, you look really fat, and they make your backside look huge'*.

> ▶ If your friend had got a C grade in a test and said, *'I will never be able to do this work. I am an idiot'*. You probably wouldn't say, *'Yes, you are really stupid, and you always get things wrong'*.

> ▶ If your friend had been dumped and said, *'I am a loser. I'll never meet anyone else'*. You probably wouldn't say, *'Yes, you are a loser. No one will ever want to go out with you'*.

You would probably be

> ▶ **concerned**

> ▶ **try to comfort them**

> ▶ say **kind things**

> ▶ and try to **cheer them up**

When you notice your critical inner voice, **write down what you are thinking and saying about yourself**. It may feel odd or embarrassing to do this, but write down exactly what your critical inner voice is saying.

- ▶ **Wait** a short time and then look again at what you have written.

- ▶ Ask yourself **what you would say to your friend** if you heard them thinking and saying these things.

- ▶ Now treat yourself the same way. **Write a kinder** and less-critical message to yourself.

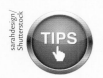

Instead of listening to your critical inner voice try to **be kinder to yourself**. Treat yourself like you would treat your friends.

 ## Don't kick yourself when you are down

If you are feeling stressed, angry, or down, don't make it worse by blaming yourself for feeling so bad. You wouldn't blame yourself if you caught a cold. You would look after yourself and do something nice to help you feel better.

If you have had a difficult day and feel bad, don't punish or blame yourself for what has happened or how you feel. **Care for yourself** and do something to help you feel better.

- ▶ Enjoy a long relaxing bath with candles.

- ▶ Paint your nails or do your hair.

- ▶ Watch an episode of your favourite serial or box set.

- ▶ Go for a walk.

- ▶ Eat a slice of cake or a biscuit.

- ▶ Make a drink of hot chocolate.

Stop beating yourself up. You don't deserve to feel like this. Look after yourself, and **do something that will make you feel better**.

 ## Forgive mistakes

Our critical inner voice is very good at finding faults in the things we do. Instead of focusing on these and blaming ourselves for making mistakes, try to **be more forgiving**. Remember the following:

We all get things wrong. Everyone makes mistakes, so don't give yourself a hard time for getting something wrong. Expect things to go wrong. Learn from your mistakes, and plan what you will do differently next time.

We all have off days. Some days will be better than others. It is just the way it is. Try again tomorrow, and see what happens.

Be patient. It often takes time to get things right. You didn't learn to ride a bike, read a book, play music, or a sport straight away. It takes time. Celebrate what you have achieved rather than criticising yourself for what you have not yet done.

Give yourself **permission to make mistakes**. Learn from what happens, and decide what you will do differently next time.

 ## Celebrate what you achieve

We all want to do well, but often we are never satisfied with what we achieve. Our standards become too high so that we always end up failing. Instead of setting ourselves up to fail, **celebrate what you achieve**.

Stop comparing yourself against others. We tend to find the most successful person and compare ourselves against them. It is not surprising that we feel inadequate. You don't have to be better than everyone else, so stop comparing yourself to others.

You can't always be 'the best'. There will be many times when others are better at things than you. Famous celebrities may be good at acting, music, or sport, but there will be plenty of things they struggle to do. Focus on your strengths, and don't expect to be the best at everything you do.

Avoid 'should' and 'musts'. Words like these set us up to fail. When we say we 'should' or 'must' do something, we are really saying that what we have done isn't right or good enough. Recognise and value what you have achieved.

Reward effort not success. Focusing on outcomes can remind you of what you have not achieved. You probably tried to do your best, so focus on your effort not the outcome.

Each day **write down one or two of your achievements**. Over time this will grow and help you to notice and celebrate what you have achieved.

Accept who you are

We spend a lot of time thinking about our imperfections, and how we could be different. We are often dissatisfied with ourselves, and may want to be taller, slimmer, brighter, more attractive, or better at sports.

Instead of wishing you could be different, **accept and value yourself for who you are**. Focus on

Your qualities – are you patient, determined, hard-working, kind, reliable, sensitive, honest, understanding, or see things through?

Your relationships – are you a good listener, supportive, loyal, caring, trust-worthy, considerate, supportive, or a good laugh?

Your appearance – are you well proportioned, have a nice body shape, eyes, hair, skin, hands, nails, mouth, teeth, or have a nice voice?

Your skills – are you good at sport, music, school work, art, drama, gaming, cooking, singing, being creative, growing things, putting on make-up, or caring for animals?

Instead of focusing on the things you would like to change, **accept yourself for who you are**. Remind yourself that you are special, and that there is nobody else like you.

Speak kindly to yourself

Our critical inner voice is very harsh and unkind. We say things in our heads that we would find embarrassing to speak out aloud. Try to **develop a kinder inner voice** that recognises.

- How you are **feeling right now.**
- That you are **not alone** in how you feel.
- That you need to **be kind to yourself**.

Try to develop one or two short 'kind' statements that work for you.

'I am having a hard time. Everybody finds things difficult. I need to look after myself'.

'I am feeling really down. Lots of people feel like me. I need to accept myself for who I am'.

'I am really angry. We all feel angry at times. I am trying my best to cope with this'.

Repeat your kinder inner voice at the start and end of each day. Stand in front of a mirror and say it out aloud in a kind voice.

 Find the good in others

When we feel anxious, angry, or down, it often feels that

▸ everyone is **picking on you**

▸ as if the world is **out to get you**

▸ that these things **only happen to you**

▸ that everyone is **mean or unkind**

Because you are expecting people to be unkind, you are probably looking for evidence of this. The more you look, the more you will probably find.

Try to change this by looking for the times that someone has been caring or considerate. **Assume the best in people and enjoy kindness**. Look for those times when someone

▸ makes time to talk and listen to someone

▸ says something nice. It can be as simple as 'I like your trainers' or 'you hair looks good'

▸ is caring and ask someone if they are feeling alright or gives someone a hug or makes them a drink

▸ helps out by doing a chore like laying the table, cooking a meal, or doing the washing up

▸ shares something like their music or chocolate

▸ sends a nice email or text

▸ says thank you to a friend, bus driver, your teacher, or parent

▸ makes someone laugh or smile

Try to find one example each day **where someone has been kind**. You might find that people are kinder than you thought.

Be kind to others

You know how good it feels when people are kind to you, so why don't you make an extra effort to **be kind to someone else**. Give a compliment, smile, offer to help, or take time to listen to what they have to say.

At the end of each day write down any of your acts of kindness and plan, what you could do tomorrow **to be kind to someone**.

ValentinT / Shutterstock

Our inner voice can be harsh, critical, and very unkind.

Rather than beating ourselves up we need to accept that

▶ things will go wrong

▶ we are not perfect

▶ we will make mistakes

▶ unkind things happen.

Don't tear yourself apart. Learn to be kind to yourself, be kind to others, and accept yourself for who you are.

Treat yourself like a friend

We are often very unkind and critical of ourselves. We treat ourselves very differently to how we would treat our friends. When you notice your 'inner critic' write down exactly what you are thinking and calling yourself. Wait for a short time and look at what you have written.

▶ Ask yourself what you would say to your friend if you heard them thinking and saying these things.

▶ Now treat yourself the same way, and write a kinder message to yourself.

What am I thinking and calling myself?

What would I say to my friends if I heard them saying this?

What should I say to myself now?

Look after yourself

When you feel down don't beat yourself up or blame yourself for feeling so bad. Look after yourself.

Make a list of all the treats that make you feel better.

▶ Long bath, washing your hair, putting on your make-up, or painting your nails.

▶ Watching a DVD, going for a walk, or sitting in the park.

▶ Eating a slice of toast, cake or biscuit, or drinking hot chocolate.

Treats that make me feel better

When you are feeling down or had a bad day, look after yourself. Choose something to make yourself feel better.

A kinder inner voice

Our inner critical voice is very harsh and unkind. Try to practice talking to yourself in a kinder less-critical way. Think about some short statements that recognise

▶ How you are feeling right now

▶ That you are not alone in how you feel

▶ That you need to be kind to yourself

'I am having a hard time. Everybody finds things difficult. I need to look after myself.'

My kinder voice

My kinder voice

My kinder voice

Stand in front of a mirror and repeat your kinder voice out aloud at the start and end of each day. Practice repeating it with kindness and confidence.

Finding kindness

Spend a few minutes each day to think about what has happened and find at least one example where

▶ someone has been kind to you, or

▶ you have been kind to someone else

Day	What happened

Looking for kindness will help you to feel better about yourself, and the people around you.

Be mindful

We spend a lot of time thinking. Thoughts are constantly racing through our minds. They provide a running commentary about what is going on, how we see ourselves, how we expect others to treat us, and what we expect will happen in the future.

Having these sorts of thoughts is not a problem. Everybody has them. The problem is that some people get **upset** by them. They spend a lot of time listening, believing, and **arguing with their thoughts**. They **over think** situations and spend lots of time **rehearsing** what has happened and **worrying** about what will happen.

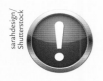

Because we are so busy thinking about the past or worrying about the future, **we don't notice what is happening right now**.

Think about what you have done today.

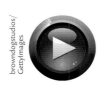

Did you really notice how you washed this morning? The smell of the soap; the sound of running water; the temperature and feel of the water on your face; the sight of the soapy bubbles; the taste of the toothpaste; the bristles of your toothbrush rubbing against your gums?

Did you really notice how you made and ate your breakfast? How you put the bread in the toaster; the smell of the toast as it cooked; the crunchy sound as you bit into it; the feeling in your fingers as you held it; the different colours on the toast; and the taste as you ate it?

Did you really notice how you walked to college or work? The smell as you walked down the road; the sounds of cars, birds, people talking; the feeling in your feet as you took each step; the different coloured doors you walked past, the feel of your bag hung over your shoulder?

Thinking Good, Feeling Better: A Cognitive Behavioural Therapy Workbook for Adolescents and Young Adults, First Edition. Paul Stallard.
© 2019 John Wiley & Sons Ltd. Published 2019 by John Wiley & Sons Ltd.
Companion website: www.wiley.com/go/thinkinggood

We do many things throughout our day, but often **our mind is somewhere else**. We are busy thinking about what has happened or worrying about what will happen rather than enjoying what is happening right here and now.

Most of our unhappiness, stress, and anger comes from thinking about the past or future. **Focusing your attention on what is happening here and now** can help you to feel better.

Mindfulness

This is a way of paying attention to what you are doing **here and now**. It is about noticing the sights, smells, sounds, and tastes that you experience. It is about observing your thoughts and feelings in a curious, open-minded, non-judgemental way.

Each letter of the word **FOCUS** can help us to remember the key steps involved in mindfulness

▶ **F**ocus your attention

▶ **O**bserve what is happening

▶ Be **C**urious

▶ **U**se your senses

▶ **S**uspend judgement

Learning to focus your attention on what is going on here and now can help you to get rid of the clutter in your head.

Focus, observe, be curious, and use your senses

We are often busy thinking and don't really notice what we are doing. We wash, eat, and move around, but often our mind is elsewhere, going over what we did or planning what we will do.

The first step of mindfulness is to learn to **focus your attention**.

▶ This is like training an active and curious puppy. Puppies like to run around and explore everything they see and will not sit quietly by your side.

> Our attention is the same. If we don't focus our attention on what we are doing, our mind will wander, and we will think about other things.

> If a puppy wanders off, we call it back. We need to do the same with our attention. As soon as you notice your attention wandering, steer it back to what is happening here and now.

Focus on what is going on around you, and **observe** what is happening.

> Imagine that you are looking through a camera with a **big zoom lens**.

> Before you look through the camera, you will find many different things to focus on.

> As you look through the camera your attention becomes more focused. You no longer see everything, but you see smaller things in more detail.

> As you zoom the camera lens in you, become more focused and notice smaller and smaller details.

Be **curious** and **use all of your sense** to explore what is happening.

> Imagine it is the very first time, you have ever seen these things.

> Use all of your senses to become more aware of the smells, sounds, feelings, sights, and tastes of the things around you.

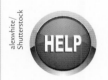

As you learn to be mindful, you will probably notice you mind wandering. This is perfectly normal. You are not doing anything wrong. The idea of mindfulness is **train your attention** and this may take a little time. Simply notice what is happening, and bring your attention back to the here and now.

Mindful breathing

Focusing on your breathing is a good way to start to learn mindfulness. You are always breathing, so this can be done anywhere without people knowing what you are doing.

Choose a quiet time when you will not be disturbed for one to two minutes. Sit comfortably with your hands on your chest. You may want to shut your eyes, but that is up to you. Now **focus your attention** and **observe your breathing**.

▶ Breathe slowly in through your nose and out through your mouth.

▶ Be **curious** and zoom in on your chest. Notice how your chest rises and falls as you breathe in and out.

▶ Feel the muscles in your chest tense and relax with each breath.

▶ Listen to the sound of your breath.

▶ Feel the cold air in your nose as you breathe in and the warm air in your mouth as you breathe out.

▶ Count 1 as you breathe in and 2 as you breathe out.

▶ Count up to 10.

▶ Don't worry if you notice your mind wandering. As soon as you become aware that your mind is not focused on your breathing, steer your attention back and count your breaths.

▶ Once you have counted to 10, start again, and enjoy this calm feeling for one to two minutes.

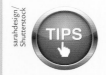

sarahdesign / Shutterstock

If you are worrying or rehearsing things, bring your mind back to the here and now, and **try mindful breathing**.

Mindful eating

We are often rushing around and don't really notice many of the everyday things we do. Try this exercise to help you focus your attention on your eating.

Choose something you enjoy eating like a piece of chocolate or fruit. **Focus your attention** and **observe it**. Hold it in your hand and look closely at it. **Be curious.** Imagine it is the very first time you have ever seen it, and **use all of your senses** to explore it:

▶ Zoom your attention in on what it **looks** like. What shape and colour is it? Is it shiny or dull?

▶ Zoom your attention in on what it **smells** like. Does it smell? Is it sweet or is it sour?

▶ Zoom your attention in on what it **feels** like. Is it hard or soft? Is it crumbly? Is it changing as you hold it?

- Put it in your mouth, but do not eat it. Does it feel big or small in your mouth? Is it juicy or dry? Is it resting on your tongue or in the corner of your mouth?

- Hold it in your month and zoom your attention in on what it **tastes** like. Is it sweet, sour, or sharp? Is there more than one flavour?

- Zoom your attention in on the sounds you **hear** as you eat. Is there a crunch as you take each bite? Is it loud or quiet? Do the sounds change as you chew?

Build mindful eating into your daily routine. At the start of each meal, be mindful of the first few mouthfuls of food. Focus your attention on the texture, taste, smell and sight of the food, and the sounds you hear as you eat.

Mindful activity

You don't have to sit still to be mindful. The idea is to focus your attention on the here and now. If you are doing something active, you can still be mindful.

One activity we do every day is walking. We often use this as a way of getting somewhere and usually spend the time rehearsing or going over worries and don't notice what is happening. **Try walking mindfully**.

- Stand upright and **focus your attention** on the weight of your body on your feet.

- As you take a step zoom your attention on to your feet

- Notice how you lift one foot, whilst the other stays on the ground.

- Notice the pressure on the bottom of your foot. How your foot presses against your shoe or sock.

- Notice how your foot becomes lighter as you lift it.

- Notice the feel of the ground beneath your shoe.

- Move your attention away from your feet and zoom in with your senses.

- **Observe** your surroundings. Zoom in on what you see. As you walk, focus on an object, and notice the colours, shapes, size, and patterns.

- **Be curious. Use your senses**. Zoom in on what you hear. Focus on the sounds of the wind, the rain, the birds, and the cars.

Zoom in on what you feel. Focus on the hot or cold feeling on your face, your bag feeling heavy on your shoulder, and the rough stones beneath your feet.

 Zoom in on what you smell. The damp smell from the rain, the sweet smell of the flowers, and the smell of food cooking.

 If you notice your mind wandering off don't worry. Guide your attention back.

 Try to do one activity each day mindfully. Focus you attention on what you are doing – how you get out of bed, take a drink from the fridge, make a sandwich, get dressed, or check your phone.

 ## *Mindful observation*

We often don't really notice many of the everyday things we use or see. Try drawing a picture of your TV controller, phone, or laptop. Now have a close look at them and see how much detail you have missed.

Select one thing each day and focus all of your attention on mindfully observing it for one minute. Take **familiar objects** like

 Your pen.

 Your phone.

 A cup or plate.

 The T-shirt you put on.

 The room you are in.

 The bus or train you are travelling on.

 The tree outside your window.

 The park or road you walk down.

 Mindfully focusing you attention on everyday objects is a quick and helpful way of attending to the here and now.

Suspend judgement

We spend a great deal of **time in our heads over thinking**. We rehearse things that have happened and worry about what might happen. We end up believing or arguing with our thoughts as if they are some sort of reality which has control over us. Our minds become cluttered as our thoughts and worries take over.

Mindfulness can help us develop a different relationship with our thoughts. We can learn to stand back from them and understand our thoughts as mental activity and our feelings as body sensations. We can learn to **suspend judgement** about their content and to let our thoughts come and go rather than arguing or engaging with them.

- You don't have to try to stop your thoughts. Let them come and go.

- You don't need to argue with them.

- They are not 'facts' or 'truths', they are thoughts and feelings.

- They are not 'evidence' that you are bad.

- They are not 'evidence' that you are wrong.

- They are thoughts and feelings which will come and go like clouds in the sky or waves on the beach.

- As one passes another arrives.

- Be curious and suspend judgement. Notice them for what they are. They are thoughts and feelings which do not control you.

- Stand back from your thoughts and feelings and observe them.

 Let your thoughts come and go. Don't try and stop them, don't argue with them, **accept them** for what they are – **mental events and body sensations**.

Mindful thinking

Once you can focus you attention on the here and now, you can use the same idea to focus on your thoughts and feelings. By curiously observing your thoughts, you will discover that you create them and that they come and go. You will notice that your thoughts effect how you feel. You don't need to stop your thoughts or change your feelings. Notice **your thoughts** and be aware of them.

Sit in a quiet place and put your hands gently on your chest. Start off by focusing all of your attention on your breathing for one minute.

▶ Zoom your attention in and focus on your thoughts.

▶ Notice how your thoughts come and go.

▶ They are like waves breaking on the beach. As one crashes another follows.

▶ They are like clouds floating in the sky. As one drifts past another follows.

▶ Imagine each wave or cloud as a thought or a feeling.

▶ As each wave or cloud comes, notice the thought or feeling.

▶ Watch it disappear as the wave crashes and the cloud drifts by.

▶ Notice the thought or feeling on the next wave or cloud and watch it disappear.

▶ **Suspend judgement**. You don't need to argue or react to them. They will pass.

▶ You don't have to try and stop them or change them. Let them come.

▶ Simply observe them.

Practice observing your thoughts and feelings each day. Notice them for what they are – the activity of your brain and the sensations of your body. They are not facts. You do not need to believe or argue with them. Suspend judgement. Observe them come and go.

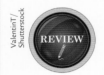

ValentinT / Shutterstock

We spend a lot of time in our heads. We worry about what will happen or rehearse what has happened. We don't pay attention to what is happening here and now.

Focus you attention, observe what is happening, be curious, and use your senses. Learn to suspend judgement and recognise your thoughts as activity of your brain.

Your thoughts will come and go. You don't need to stop or argue with them. They are not 'facts', and they do not control you.

Mindful breathing

You can use this short exercise as many times as you like throughout the day. It is a useful way of focusing your attention on the here and now.

- ▷ Choose a quiet place where you will not be disturbed for one to two minutes.

- ▷ Sit comfortably with your hands resting gently on your chest.

- ▷ Breathe slowly in through your nose and out through your mouth.

- ▷ Notice how your chest rises and falls as you breathe in and out.

- ▷ Feel the muscles in your chest tense and relax with each breath.

- ▷ Listen to the sound of your breath.

- ▷ Feel the cold air in your nose as you breathe in and the warm air in your mouth as you breathe out.

- ▷ Count 1 as you breathe in and 2 as you breathe out.

- ▷ Count up to 10 and enjoy this calm feeling.

Don't worry if you mind wanders. As soon as you notice it, bring your attention back to your breathing.

Mindful thinking

Sometimes our minds feel cluttered with a constant stream of thoughts and worries. We end up thinking about what has happened or worrying about what will happen and don't notice what is happening here and now.

▶ Choose a quiet place where you will not be disturbed.

▶ Start by focusing all your attention on your breathing.

▶ After a minute, zoom your attention onto the thoughts tumbling through your head.

▶ Notice how your thoughts come and go.

▶ They are like waves breaking on the beach. As one crashes another follows.

▶ They are like clouds floating in the sky. As one drifts past another follows.

▶ Imagine each wave or cloud as a thought or a feeling.

▶ As each wave or cloud comes, be curious and notice the thought or feeling.

▶ Watch it disappear as the wave crashes and the cloud drifts by.

▶ Notice the thought or feeling on the next wave or cloud and watch it disappear.

▶ You don't need to argue or react with them. They will pass.

▶ Simply observe them.

Mindful observation

Identify one thing each day that usually goes un-noticed or unappreciated. It could be

▶ everyday objects like a pen, plate, mug, pair of jeans, or a flower.

▶ familiar places like your bedroom wall, a drawer in the kitchen, or a picture hanging on the wall.

▶ objects we often use like a phone, computer, TV or book.

Focus **all your attention** on your chosen object for one minute and examine it very carefully.

Day	What I observed

Do I really notice what I use?

We take many everyday objects for granted. We turn on the TV, send messages on our phones, and search the Internet, but don't really notice the TV controller, phone, or computer keyboard we use.

Try drawing a picture of an everyday object. It could be anything like the TV controller, your phone, breakfast cereal box, or coffee jar. Draw it from memory and draw it in as much detail as possible.

Now look at your object. Observe it closely. Use another coloured pen and add the parts that you missed to your drawing.

Getting ready to change

Life can be full of problems. Parents, friends, boy/girlfriends, college, and work; in fact almost everything creates problems at some stage or another.

▶ You **might be criticised** by your family.

▶ Your friends **might be unkind** or leave you out of their plans.

▶ You **may not understand** your work.

▶ You may have to do something you have **never done before**.

We are quite **good at coping** with many of our problems, and they are quickly sorted out. Other problems can be harder to sort out. They might

▶ happen **fairly often**

▶ have been around for a **long time**

▶ seem **overwhelming**

▶ **limit what you do**

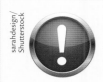

When problems take over, we **feel** worried, stressed, angry, or unhappy.

These feelings are common and often pass, but sometimes they **become very strong**:

▶ Life becomes **one big worry**.

▶ We feel anxious or **stressed all the time**.

▶ We feel sad or unhappy and **never have any happy days**.

▶ We **feel angry and irritable** and seem to be always arguing.

Thinking Good, Feeling Better: A Cognitive Behavioural Therapy Workbook for Adolescents and Young Adults, First Edition. Paul Stallard.
© 2019 John Wiley & Sons Ltd. Published 2019 by John Wiley & Sons Ltd.
Companion website: www.wiley.com/go/thinkinggood

When we **feel** worried, stressed, angry, or unhappy, we **may not want to do things**.

We might

▶ **make excuses** and put things off

▶ **avoid** the things that make us worry or feel anxious

▶ find it **hard to motivate** ourselves

▶ **stop trying** so hard

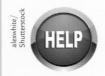

alexwhite/
Shutterstock

We need to **understand** why this happens, and how you can **feel better** and **regain your life**.

One way of helping is called **Cognitive Behaviour Therapy (CBT)**. This helps us to understand the way we think about things and the effect of this on how we feel and what we do.

What you think

When we do something, there will be many different thoughts rushing around our heads. We don't always notice these thoughts, but they are usually there.

There will be times when our thoughts seem very loud. If we are feeling anxious, angry, or low in our mood, these thoughts are often **unhelpful**. They are

▶ **very negative** and focus on what might go wrong – *'I don't know what to talk about and everyone will laugh at me'*.

▶ **very critical** of you and how you behave – *'I'm stupid and always get my work wrong'*.

▶ **talk you out of doing things** or trying so hard – *'No one likes me, so I might as well stay at home'*.

How you feel

We experience many different emotions every day. Some are short-lived, some make sense, and others seem to last and take over.

Unhelpful ways of thinking make us **feel unpleasant**, and we might feel anxious, angry, or unhappy.

▶ If you **think** that you don't know what to talk about, you might **feel** anxious.

▶ If you **think** that you will get your work wrong, you might **feel** angry.

▶ If you **think** that your friends do not like, you may **feel** sad.

What you do

What you think and how you feel will have an effect on what you do. Unhelpful thoughts and unpleasant feelings may make you **stop**, **give up**, or **avoid** doing things.

▶ If you **think** you don't know what to say to your friends, you might **avoid** talking when you are with them.

▶ If you **think** you will get your work wrong, you might **give up** and not bother trying.

▶ If you **think** that you are not liked by your friends, you might **stop** going out and stay at home on your own.

The negative trap

Because of the connection between what we think, how we feel, and what we do, we can end up stuck in a **negative trap**.

Unhelpful ways of thinking make us **feel unpleasant** and **stop us** from doing things.

We now **behave in ways that confirm our thinking**. As if by magic, our unhelpful thoughts have come true.

▶ Because you don't say much when you are with your friends, you will worry even more that *'they think I've got nothing to say, and won't want to hang out with me'*.

▶ Because you don't try with your work, you might get things wrong and think *'I knew I was stupid'*.

▶ Because you don't go out with you friends, you might stay at home and think *'I knew no one liked me. I am home on my own again'*.

We all fall into this negative trap at times, but some people become stuck.

▶ Their thoughts are **often unhelpful**.

▶ They feel **unpleasant most of the time**.

▶ They end up doing **fewer of the things they would like to do**.

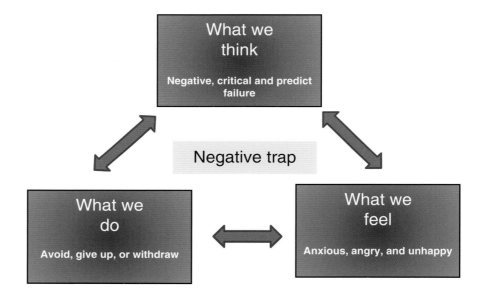

Good news

If we can understand more about the way we think, we might be able to discover ways in which we can help ourselves to feel better and to cope with problems and challenges.

We can do this by testing the way we think so that we can **develop more helpful and balanced ways of thinking**. This will help us discover that

▶ things might go wrong, but they are often **not as bad** as you think they will be

▶ **you do cope**, but often overlook or downplay these times

▶ **you can do** something to change how you feel and regain control of your life.

RFvectors / Shutterstock

Are you ready to try?

Living with your problems is hard. They stop you from doing the things you would like to do. You would probably like things to be different, but trying to change isn't always easy. To change things you will need to

Be open to new ideas: Some ideas may seem odd, but you may be surprised how helpful they can be. Be open to new ideas and don't dismiss them.

Try doing things differently: Often you have to experiment with doing things differently and to practice new skills and ways of coping. Nothing works/helps every time so give it a go and try each new idea a few times.

Be Positive: Challenges and worries can feel overwhelming, but keep positive and see what you can do to help yourself feel better.

Thinking Good, Feeling Better works best when you are feeling motivated and believe that you can make a difference to the way you feel. If you are unsure, then these ideas probably won't be so helpful. It may be better to wait until you feel more motivated.

My goals

If you are ready to try to change, the next job is to work out your **goals**. How do you want things to be different? What do you want to be able to do?

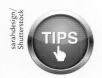

sarahdesign / Shutterstock

Setting yourself goals helps you to **focus on the future**. They will remind you what you want to achieve and help you to keep track of the **progress you are making**.

The best goals are **SMART** goals:

Specific – clearly and positively define what you want to do. Instead of setting a goal 'to get fit' be specific – 'I will join a gym and train twice a week'.

Measurable – it is important to choose a goal you can measure so that you can check how you are doing. So instead of 'I will be more sociable', your goal could be that 'I will eat my lunch with people on two days this week'.

Achievable – goals should be motivating. If they are too large, they may feel impossible. If you are struggling to even get out of bed, then a goal of 'going out with friends for one hour everyday' will feel impossible. Make sure your goal is achievable.

Relevant – choose goals that are important to you. If you want to go out more often, there is no point in choosing a goal 'to go to the local supermarket' unless it is something you really want to do. You need to feel pleased and proud of what you have done.

Timely – make sure you can achieve your goal within a reasonable time. If it takes too long, you may become frustrated and feel that you are not making any progress. It is better to choose smaller goals that you can achieve quicker.

SMART goals focus on what you want to achieve. Once you have chosen your goals, **rate them each week** between 1 (no progress) and 10 (totally achieved) to see how much progress you are making.

The miracle question

Another way of discovering your goals is to ask yourself the '**miracle question**'. Instead of focusing on your problems in the here and now, the miracle question asks you to think about the **future** and how you and your life would be different if you no longer had any problems. The miracle question might be like this:

Imagine that overnight a miracle happens, and you wake in the morning to find that all your problems have gone.

▶ How will **you feel?**

▶ What will **you be doing?**

▶ How will you **be thinking** about yourself and what you do?

▶ How will **other people know** that things have changed?

TIPS

Think about the **future**, and how you would like things to be different. Now think of the steps you can take to make that happen.

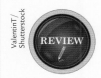

ValentinT/ Shutterstock

REVIEW

We can end up thinking in unhelpful ways which make us feel unpleasant and stop us from doing things. This is the negative trap.

We need to understand how this happens so that we can break out of this trap.

Think about how you would like things to be different and set yourself some goals.

Are you ready to change?

You can check whether you are ready to change by choosing a number from 1 to 100 to show how much you believe the questions. Below

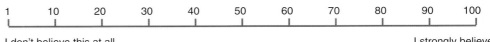

| 1 | 10 | 20 | 30 | 40 | 50 | 60 | 70 | 80 | 90 | 100 |

I don't believe this at all   I strongly believe this

It is possible to do something about my problems

I can beat my problems

I think this way of working (CBT) will help me

I will be able to change things

This is the right time to try and change things

> What might get in the way or stop you from making these changes?

If you score 50 or less on any of these questions, you may want to talk with someone about whether this is the right time to try and change things.

Cognitive behaviour therapy

What is cognitive behaviour therapy (CBT)?

CBT helps to understand the link between what we think, how we feel, and what we do.

Why is this link important?

People often think in negative, critical, or unhelpful ways that make them feel anxious, angry, or unhappy.

When we feel like this, we find it hard to do things. The less we do, the more we think, and the worse we feel.

How can CBT change this?

CBT will help you find more helpful and balanced ways of thinking and how to control your unpleasant feelings. It will help you reclaim your life, so that you can do the things you really want to do.

Will it help me?

CBT is a very effective way of helping young people deal with problems and cope with challenges. We don't know for sure whether it will help you, but you may find some of the ideas useful.

What happens in CBT?

We will work together to understand the way you think and experiment with different ideas to find out what helps you feel better and to do the things you want to do.

The miracle question

Imagine that a miracle happens overnight. When you wake up in the morning, all your problems have gone.

How will you feel?

What will you be able to do?

How will you be thinking?

How will other people know that things are different?

What small steps will take you to your problem-free future?

1.

2.

3.

My goals

It is helpful to set yourself some goals. These will remind you what you want to achieve and how much progress you are making. Make sure you have **SMART** goals and choose a number between 1 and 100 to rate your progress each week.

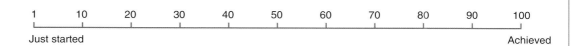

1   10   20   30   40   50   60   70   80   90   100

Just started   Achieved

My goals	How am I doing?									
	Week 1	Week 2	Week 3	Week 4	Week 5	Week 6	Week 7	Week 8	Week 9	Week 10
1.										
2.										
3.										

Thoughts, feelings, and what you do

Cognitive behaviour therapy or CBT helps to understand the link between **what we think, how we feel, and what we do**.

Thinking in negative, critical, or unhelpful ways can make us feel sad, anxious, or angry.

When we **feel** sad, anxious, or angry, we often find it hard to do things or cope with challenges.

The **less we do**, the more time we have to think and the worse we feel.

Sometimes we might get stuck in a **negative trap** where our thinking is very negative and unhelpful. We all fall into this at times, but some people get stuck and can't find a way out.

By questioning and challenging the way we think we can

▶ Develop more **positive, balanced, and helpful ways of thinking**

▶ This helps us to **feel happier, less worried, and calmer**

▶ When we feel like this, we are **more motivated** to do things and better able to face and cope with problems and challenges.

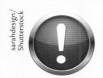

Understanding the link between what we think, how we feel, and what we do can help to get us out of the negative trap.

Thinking Good, Feeling Better: A Cognitive Behavioural Therapy Workbook for Adolescents and Young Adults, First Edition.
Paul Stallard.
© 2019 John Wiley & Sons Ltd. Published 2019 by John Wiley & Sons Ltd.
Companion website: www.wiley.com/go/thinkinggood

How does the negative trap happen?

The way we think develops over time and is shaped by some of the **important things that happen** in our lives.

▶ If you have had lots of illnesses or accidents, you might think *'bad things happen to me'*.

▶ If you have been bullied or don't have many friends you might think *'people don't like me'*.

▶ If you are often criticised or told off, you might think *'I am a failure'*.

Core beliefs

Important events can lead us to develop some very strong ways of thinking called **core beliefs**. These are **fixed, rigid, inflexible ways of thinking** about

▶ **Ourselves**, *'I am kind'*.

▶ **What we do**, *'I always get things wrong'*.

▶ **How we expect to be treated**, *'People don't like me'*.

▶ **The future**, *'I will be successful'*.

Core beliefs are often very short statements which we apply to all the situations we encounter.

Assumptions

Core beliefs can be **helpful** and help us to make sense of our lives. They help us to predict, or make assumptions, about what will happen and how others will behave. We think that **if** something happens, **then** something will follow.

▶ If *'I am kind'*, **then** other people will like me.

▶ If *'I work hard'*, **then** I will get good exam grades.

▶ **If** *'people are out to get me'*, **then** people can not be trusted.

▶ **If** *'I will be successful'*, **then** I will get a good job.

 Beliefs and assumptions can be **helpful**. They **motivate** us to do things, encourage us to face our challenges, and make us **feel good**.

Unhelpful beliefs

Sometimes our core beliefs can be **unhelpful**. Beliefs like *'I must be perfect'*, *'I am a failure'*, or *'No on loves me'* might lead us to

▶ make **false predictions**

▶ **set us up to fail**

▶ make us **feel bad**

▶ **limit what we do**

▶ **talk us out** of doing things

A belief that *'I must be perfect'* may lead you to assume that your work is never good enough. This may make you feel stressed or unhappy as you keep going over you work time and time again.

A belief that *'I am a failure'* may lead you to assume that there is no point trying with your schoolwork. You may feel sad and end up in trouble at school for not handing in your work.

A belief that *'No one loves me'* may make you assume that other people will be unkind to you. You may feel sad or worried and spend lots of time on your own.

 Beliefs and assumptions can be unhelpful. They make us less motivated to face our challenges and make us feel unpleasant.

Beliefs are strong

Core beliefs are very strong and powerful ways of thinking which are resistant to any challenge. We keep them strong in two main ways:

We constantly look for evidence, no matter how small, as proof that they are right.

▶ Your mum might have had a really busy day and not had a chance to wash that special item of clothing you wanted to wear. You might see this as evidence that *'no one cares about me'*.

We ignore or dismiss as unimportant anything that questions them.

▶ If you had a belief that *'No one likes me'*, you might reject any positive comments from your parents as *'they don't really mean that'*.

Turning your beliefs on

We will have a number of core beliefs. They are like a series of light switches. They are always there, but they get turned on and come to the front of our thinking at certain times.

Core beliefs are turned on by events similar to those that created them:

▶ Being asked to complete your work may turn on your core belief that *'you must be perfect'*.

▶ Failing your driving test may turn on your core belief *'that I always fail'*.

▶ Being dropped by your boyfriend or girlfriend may turn on your core belief that *'No one loves me'*.

Automatic thoughts

Once turned on, our core beliefs and assumptions produce lots of thoughts. These are **automatic thoughts**. They tumble through our heads providing a running commentary about what is going on.

These are the thoughts we notice most. We often notice them when we are unoccupied. If our beliefs and assumptions are unhelpful, our automatic thoughts will be negative and critical.

Negative thoughts focus on what might go wrong:
'I don't know what to talk about and everyone will laugh at me'.

Critical thoughts criticise you and how you behave:
'I'm stupid and always get my school work wrong'.

Unhelpful thoughts talk you out of doing things or coping:
'No one likes me, so I might as well stay at home'.

▶ Being asked to complete your work may trigger negative automatic thoughts like *'I don't know what to do', 'This isn't good enough',* or *'I am sure this is wrong'.*

▶ Failing your driving test may result in negative automatic thoughts like *'I really screwed this up', 'I'll never be able to drive'* and *'That examiner didn't like me'.*

▶ A relationship ending may result in negative automatic thoughts like *'I knew this wouldn't last, it never does', 'He/she is making fun of me'* and *'I'll never have another relationship'.*

How you feel

How you think will affect how you feel.

Positive or helpful thoughts make you **feel good**:

▶ If you thought *'I am really looking forward to my party'*, you would probably feel excited.

▶ If you thought *'I look good in these clothes'*, you would probably feel happy.

▶ If you thought *'I know how to do this'*, you would probably feel relaxed.

Negative or critical thoughts make you **feel unpleasant**:

▶ If you thought *'No one will turn up to my party'*, you would probably feel anxious.

▶ If you thought *'These clothes don't fit'*, you might feel unhappy.

▶ If you thought *'I don't know how to do this'*, you might feel angry or stressed.

Many of these feelings will not be very strong and will quickly pass. In fact you may not even notice them.

At other times, these unpleasant feelings take over. They might become very strong or seem to last as you end up feeling constantly stressed, unhappy, or angry.

What you do

When these feelings last or become very strong, they start to have an effect on what we do. We want to feel good, so we try to do more of those things that make us feel good and less of those things that make us feel unpleasant

If we **feel unpleasant** we might

▶ **Stop** doing things

▶ **Avoid** situations that might be difficult

▶ **Give up** trying to do things

If you feel angry when your work is criticised, you may **stop** going to work or college. You may feel calmer when you stay at home.

If you feel anxious when talking with other people, you may **avoid** going out. You may feel more relaxed staying at home or being on your own.

If you feel sad and unhappy, you may not have much energy to do things. You may feel unmotivated and **give up** doing things you used to enjoy.

The negative trap

The less you do, the more time you spend on your own, and the more you hear your unhelpful thoughts.

Because your beliefs are very strong and you hear your thoughts so often, you **look for evidence** which proves that your **thoughts were right** all along.

▶ Receiving a call from college asking for a meeting to discuss your attendance may prove the thought *'they just want to have a go at me'*.

▶ Staying at home on your own could prove the thought that *'I have no friends'*.

▶ Not going to training with your sports club could prove the thought *'I can't do anything'*.

This is the **negative trap** where your thoughts seem to magically become true. Let us check this again because often we only look for evidence to support our negative thoughts and ignore or dismiss anything that challenges them. We only see one side of the story, so check whether there is something you have overlooked?

▶ You may have overlooked that college said they wanted to find a way to help you get back to your lessons.

▶ You may have overlooked the texts from your friend asking if you wanted to do something at the weekend.

▶ You may have forgotten that you have not been feeling very well today but did go training last week.

You can break out of the negative trap. Learn to **develop more helpful and balanced ways of thinking** that make you feel better and help you to do the things you really want to do.

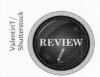

Valentin T /
Shutterstock

We may fall into a negative trap where we think in ways that make us feel unpleasant and stop us from doing things.

We need to understand the way we think, how we feel, and what we do.

Developing more balanced and helpful ways of thinking will make us feel better and encourage us to do things.

The negative trap

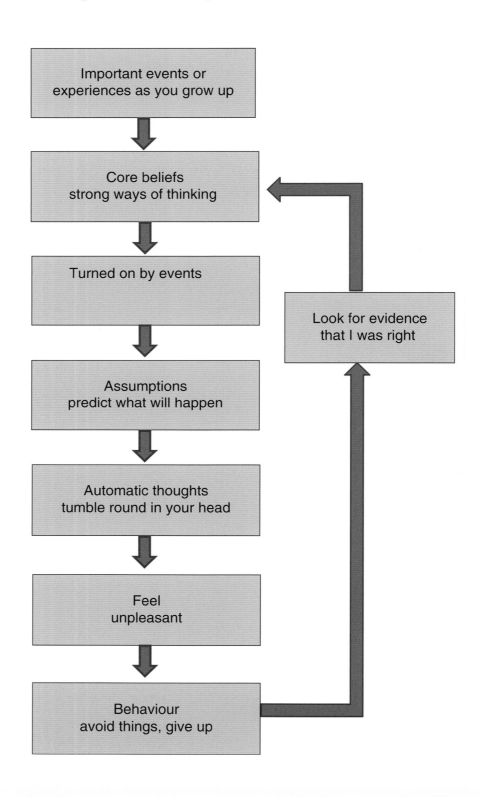

Important events or
experiences as you grow up

↓

Core beliefs
strong ways of thinking

↓

Turned on by events

↓

Assumptions
predict what will happen

↓

Automatic thoughts
tumble round in your head

↓

Feel
unpleasant

↓

Behaviour
avoid things, give up

Look for evidence
that I was right

Unhelpful thoughts

Think about a situation you find difficult and write down

▶ what the situation is

▶ the thoughts you notice tumbling around your head

▶ the feelings and body signals you notice

▶ what you end up doing

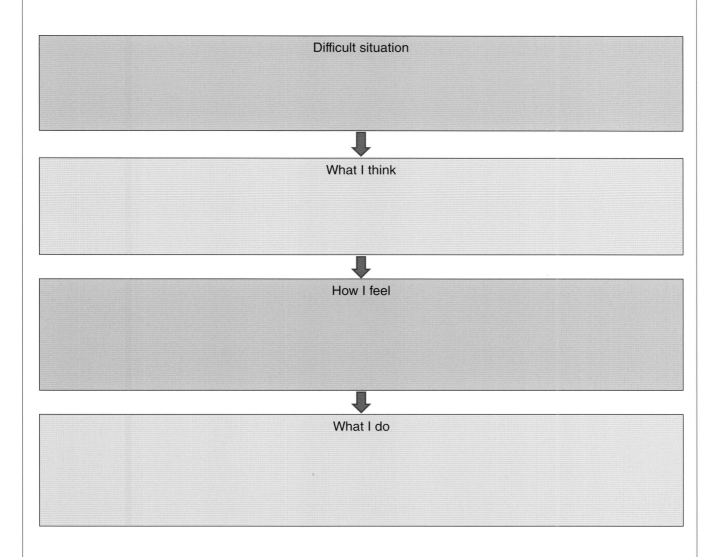

THE WAY YOU THINK

CHAPTER NINE

The way you think

We have a constant stream of thoughts running through our mind. They provide a commentary about what has happened, what we are doing, and what we will do.

Imagine that you have been invited to a party. All your friends are going. You are going to stay late, and there is going to be great music. As you get ready for the party, you might notice yourself **thinking**:

▶ *'I am going to look great in these clothes'.*

▶ *'All my friends are texting to check what time to meet'.*

▶ *'This is going to be so much fun'.*

When you **think** like this, you will probably **feel** excited or happy and will be **busy** making plans, talking with friends, and getting yourself ready.

You could find yourself thinking very differently. You may be unsure what to wear or who will be there. As you get ready you might notice yourself **thinking**:

▶ *'I look awful in these clothes'.*

▶ *'No one has called to ask what time I am going'.*

▶ *'This is going to be terrible'.*

When you **think** like this, you will probably **feel** worried or unhappy. You will probably **put off** getting ready and be unsure whether to go.

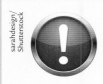

Exploring the way you think can help you to understand how you feel and how you behave.

Thinking Good, Feeling Better: A Cognitive Behavioural Therapy Workbook for Adolescents and Young Adults, First Edition. Paul Stallard.
© 2019 John Wiley & Sons Ltd. Published 2019 by John Wiley & Sons Ltd.
Companion website: www.wiley.com/go/thinkinggood

Hot thoughts

Our thoughts are there all the time, but we don't always hear them. The thoughts we notice most are those that **create strong feelings**.

These are **hot thoughts** and are usually about how you see yourself, what you do, how you expect others to treat you, and how you see your future.

How you see yourself – these are about you and how you see your strengths and skills.

▶ *'I am stupid'.*

▶ *'I am kind'.*

▶ *'I am a failure'.*

What you do – the way you assess what you do.

▶ *'I never get things right'.*

▶ *'I am good at art'.*

▶ *'I always work hard'.*

How you expect to be treated – our experiences as we grow up shape how we expect people to behave towards us.

▶ *'People don't like me'.*

▶ *'Mum and dad always help me'.*

▶ *'No one cares about me'.*

Your future – these are about the future and what you think will happen.

▶ *'I'll never be able to cope on my own'.*

▶ *'I will be successful and will go to college'.*

▶ *'I'll never have a relationship that lasts'.*

Helpful thoughts

Some ways of thinking are useful. They make us feel good and encourage us to do things. These are the **helpful** thoughts which recognise

▶ **Positive** things about us – *'My hair looks good like this'.*

- Our **strengths and successes** – '*I get on well with people, so I am sure I'll be able to make new friends*'.

- Focus on our **achievements** and the things that go well – '*I played really well in that game*'.

- Focus on **coping** and **being successful** – '*This is going to be really hard, but I am sure I can do this*'.

Helpful thoughts **motivate** and **encourage us** to face our challenges. They help us to cope and **be successful**.

Unhelpful thoughts

Other ways of thinking are less helpful. They make us feel unpleasant and stop us from doing things. These are the **unhelpful** thoughts like the following:

- **Negative** – '*My hair looks a mess*'.

- **Critical** of ourselves or what we do – '*People don't like me so no one will want to hang out with me*'.

- Focus on the things that **go wrong or** aren't right – '*I really messed that game up*'.

- Predict that we will **not cope** or be unsuccessful – '*I can't do this*'.

Unhelpful thoughts make us **put off or avoid** our challenges. They make us feel that we won't be successful and **can't cope**.

Automatic thoughts

The thoughts that tumble through our heads are called **automatic thoughts**. We all have them. They share the following features:

Automatic – they just happen. They pop up without you having to think of them.

Continuous – they are there all the time. No matter how hard you try you can't turn them off.

Reasonable – they seem to make sense. You accept them as true without challenging or questioning them.

Private – we rarely tell anyone what we are thinking. They remain private and keep tumbling around our heads.

 ## The negative trap

We will have a mix of helpful and unhelpful automatic thoughts. We often recognise the positive as well as the negative things that happen. We see the whole picture and are able to recognise our strengths and skills whilst being aware of our limitations. This is **balanced thinking**.

Sometimes we fall into a negative trap. When this happens

▶ Our thoughts become **distorted**. We only notice our **negative** and **critical** thoughts.

▶ We only hear the thoughts which focus on **failure** and the things that **go wrong**.

▶ We become convinced that we will **not cope**.

 Because we hear our negative thoughts so often, they **seem reasonable**. The more we hear them, the more we believe them and **accept them as true**.

 Sara was waiting at the bus stop when she noticed herself becoming uptight and tearful. Sara tried to catch the **hot thoughts** that were racing through her mind.

▶ **What were you thinking?**
Sara was thinking about the boy she met last night. She liked him and was looking forward to meeting him again, but Sara was worried that he wouldn't turn up.

▶ **What were you thinking about yourself?**
Sara was thinking that he *'didn't really like her'*. She *'didn't look that good last night'*, and there are *'many girls more attractive to me'*.

▶ How did you expect to be treated?

Sara was thinking about the times other people had let her down. She found herself thinking that '*He didn't seem that keen when we left*'; '*He has probably lost my telephone number, so he won't call*'.

▶ What did you think would happen?

Sara had now convinced herself that he would not turn up. She would have to explain to her friends that she had been stood up, and they would all laugh at her.

This was being acted out in Sara's mind. The more she had these thoughts, the worse she felt, and the more convinced she became that this would actually happen. It's not surprising that Sara felt so uptight and sad! It all started to make sense.

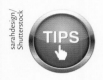

Check the way you think. When you notice a strong feeling try to find your thoughts, and see if they are helpful or unhelpful.

We have a constant stream of thoughts racing through our minds.

Sometimes these thoughts are negative, critical, and unhelpful.

Check your thoughts and see if you are thinking in unhelpful ways.

Check your thoughts

When you notice a strong emotion or some thoughts racing through your mind write them down.

> What were you thinking about yourself?

> How did you think others will treat you?

> What did you think would happen?

Are there any particular thoughts that happen more often?

Hot thoughts

When you notice a strong emotion, try to catch the thoughts that are racing through your mind.

▶ What were you doing?

▶ How did you feel?

▶ What were you thinking?

Day and time	What were you doing?	How were you feeling?	What HOT thoughts were racing through your mind?

Is the way you are thinking helpful or unhelpful?

Download your head

Don't worry if you can't find any thoughts. This sometimes happens when you go looking for them. If this happens, try downloading your head.

When you notice a change in how you are feeling write down as much as you can about what happened, who was there, what was said, and how you felt.

Write down what happened in as much detail as you can.

Read this again the next day, and underline any thoughts you managed to catch.

Thinking traps

We have found that there are ways of thinking which are helpful and others that are unhelpful.

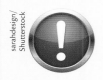

sarahdesign/
Shutterstock

Helpful thoughts make you **feel pleasant**. These are **'go' thoughts** which **encourage** you to try and do things.

▶ If you think *'I am looking forward to that party tonight'*, you may feel excited and happy and will prepare to get ready.

▶ If you think *'I have never done this before, but I will give it a go'*, you may feel calm and motivated.

▶ If you think *'I like being with Jo and Sam'*, you may feel happy and want to be with them.

Unhelpful thoughts make you **feel unpleasant**. These are **'stop' thoughts** which **talk you out** of trying to do things.

▶ If you think *'I won't know anyone at that party'*, you may feel anxious and be unsure about going.

▶ If you think *'I have never done this before and don't know what to do'*, you may feel sad and less likely to try.

▶ If you think *'Jo and Sam always leave me out'*, you may feel angry and stay on your own.

We don't chose to think in unhelpful ways. It is something we learn to do over time. We may have had some bad experiences, things may have gone wrong,

Thinking Good, Feeling Better: A Cognitive Behavioural Therapy Workbook for Adolescents and Young Adults, First Edition.
Paul Stallard.
© 2019 John Wiley & Sons Ltd. Published 2019 by John Wiley & Sons Ltd.
Companion website: www.wiley.com/go/thinkinggood

or we may have tried to do something and felt really bad afterwards. This can make us take more notice of the negative things that happen, the times we are unsuccessful and when we don't cope.

The more we focus on the negative, the more evidence we find to convince ourselves that

▶ **negative** things are always happening

▶ we **fail** at everything we do and

▶ we can **never cope** with problems.

We become caught in a **negative trap** where we overlook or dismiss the good things that happen and only see the negative.

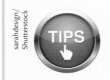

sarahdesign/Shutterstock

The first step to changing this is to become aware of the way you think and to find out about five of the common **thinking traps** that we make.

Negative filter

With this trap, we only focus on the **negative things** that happen – things that go wrong, our faults, the unkind things people say, or the times we didn't cope. Anything positive is overlooked, disbelieved, or thought to be unimportant. There are two common types of negative filters.

?RFvectors/?Shutterstock

Negative glasses

The negative glasses stop you from seeing the positive things that happen. They only let you see the negative things that occur.

▶ You may have had a really good day at college, but on the way out, you trip over. You may find yourself thinking *'I've made a fool of myself. Everyone was laughing'*. You have overlooked the rest of the day as you focus on this one event.

Positive doesn't count

With this thinking trap, you ignore or rubbish anything positive that happens. The more you do this, the more you convince yourself that only negative things happen.

> Mum or dad may have said something nice about you, but you may find yourself thinking *'They would say that because they are my parents'*.

> The person who hears that a boy or girl wants to hang out with them may think *'they probably can't find anyone else to hang out with'*.

 To counter the tendency to focus on the negative try to find the positive things that happen.

Blowing things up

The second type of thinking traps are those where negative things are blown up and **become bigger** or more important than they really are. This happens in three main ways:

 ## *Magnifying the negative*

With this thinking trap, negative events are magnified and blown up out of all proportions.

> *'I forgot his name and **everyone** was laughing at me.'*

> As you walk in a room, you may find yourself thinking that *'**Everyone** is looking and staring at me'*.

 ## *All-or-nothing thinking*

This is thinking in extremes. It is either boiling hot or freezing cold; you are perfect or a failure, and there doesn't seem to be anything in between.

> You may have a disagreement with your best friend and think to yourself *'We will never be my friends again'*.

 ## *Disaster thinking*

This is where you find yourself thinking the worse possible outcome.

> You may find yourself feeling anxious and notice that your heart is racing very fast and think, *'Oh no, I am going to have a heart attack'*.

▶ You may feel a little dizzy and think *'I'm going to pass out'*.

TIPS Blowing things up is where negative events become bigger than they really are. Try and keep things in perspective and recognise that it may not be as bad as you are making out.

Predicting failure

The third type of thinking traps are those that focus on the future and what we expect will happen. These traps often **predict failure** and make us expect the worse. This can happens in two main ways:

The fortune teller

The fortune teller knows what is going to happen . . . and it is usually bad! The fortune teller predicts that we will fail, things will go wrong, and that we won't cope. It is not surprising that this makes us anxious.

▶ You may have been invited out with your friends and find yourself thinking *'Everyone will ignore me'*. You don't know what will happen, but you are predicting the worse, and thinking like this will make you feel more anxious.

Mind reading

The mind reader knows what everyone is thinking . . . and it is usually that others are being critical or unkind about you.

▶ You may be walking home after going out with your friends and find yourself thinking *'Sean thinks my phone is rubbish'*. Sean probably didn't say this, but you seem to know what he is thinking.

TIPS Predicting failure results in us expecting that we will not be successful and that things will go wrong. Try focusing on what you can do and what will be enjoyable.

Being down on yourself

With these traps, you are very **unkind to yourself**. You call yourself names and blame yourself for everything that goes wrong. This can happen in two ways.

Dustbin labels

You attach a label to yourself and think of everything you do in this way.

'I'm a looser.'

'I'm hopeless.'

'I'm rubbish.'

Blame me

With this trap, you feel responsible for the negative things that happen, even though you have no control over them. Everything that goes wrong seems to be down to you.

▶ *'As soon as I got on the bus, it broke down.'*

▶ As you approach your friends, you hear loud voices and arguing and find yourself thinking that *'People always fall out as soon as I arrive.'* You are blaming yourself for something that you are not responsible for – they were arguing before you arrived.

 Instead of being down on yourself think what you would say to a friend if you heard them thinking like this

Setting yourself to fail

Sometimes we set ourselves **very high standards** and have **unrealistic expectations** of what we should do. Because they are so high, we never achieve them, and so we are always failing. This can happen in two main ways:

Should and must

We sometimes think and talk to ourselves in ways that are impossible for us to achieve. They make us very aware of our failings, and the things we have not done. These often start with words such as follows:

'I should'

'I must'

'I shouldn't'

'I can't'

Expecting to be perfect

With this trap, our expectations and standards are impossibly high. Because we want to be perfect all of the time, we will be devastated when we or others fall short of our impossible standards.

▶ Because you set yourself such high standards with your schoolwork, you might be really upset or angry with a B+ or if you get anything wrong.

▶ Because you expect your friends to be trustworthy and kind, you might be very upset when they let you down.

Revise your expectations. Recognise what you achieve rather than focusing on what you have been unable to do.

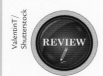

ValentinT/ Shutterstock

We can become stuck in thinking traps where we only

▶ see the negative things that happen

▶ make negative events bigger

▶ expect things to go wrong

▶ are down and unkind on ourselves

▶ have unrealistic expectations and standards

We need to get better at spotting our thinking traps. Once we know the traps we fall into, we can learn to challenge and change these to more balanced and helpful ways of thinking.

Thinking traps

Finding our thinking traps, can help us to challenge them and to develop more helpful ways of thinking. Check your thinking and write down any examples of your thinking traps.

NEGATIVE GLASSES – Can't see the positive things that happen.

POSITIVE DOESN'T COUNT – Ignore or put down anything positive.

MAGNIFYING NEGATIVES – Making small things bigger than they really are.

ALL OR NOTHING – Only think of things as extremes.

DISASTER THINKING – You imagine the worse possible outcome.

FORTUNE TELLER – You predict the worst will happen.

MIND READER – You know what everyone else is thinking.

BLAME ME – You are responsible for everything bad that happens.

DUSTBIN LABELS – You give yourself an unkind label.

EXPECTING TO BE PERFECT – Setting impossibly high standards.

SHOULD AND MUST – Failing to meet your expectations.

Thoughts and feelings

When you notice a strong feeling, write it down and describe what was happening. Try and catch any thoughts that are racing through your mind and check to see if you have fallen into a thinking trap.

Day and time	What was happening and who was there?	How did you feel?	What were you thinking?	Are you in a thinking trap? Which one?

Change your thinking

It is easy to fall into a negative way of thinking. We all do it. This is normal, but for some people, this negative, critical, and biased way of thinking takes over.

They become stuck in a **negative trap** and can only see the bad things that happen. They expect things to go wrong and think that the bad things that happen are bigger than they really are. The more we think like this, the more we believe our thoughts.

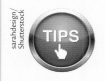

Rather than listening to your negative thoughts and accepting them as true, check them to see if there is a more helpful way of thinking using four steps – **catch it, check it, challenge it, and change it**.

Catch it

When you notice a **strong unpleasant feeling** or that you are putting off or **avoiding something**, try to catch the thoughts that are racing through you head. Are they helpful, do they make you feel good and encourage you to do things?

Write them down on a piece of paper, your laptop, phone, or PC. You may think they seem silly, but don't worry. These are the thoughts that are making you feel bad, so you need to catch and check them out.

Check it

The next step is to check your thoughts and to see whether you are **caught in a thinking trap?** Check them to see whether you are making things out to be worse than they really are.

Thinking Good, Feeling Better: A Cognitive Behavioural Therapy Workbook for Adolescents and Young Adults, First Edition. Paul Stallard.
© 2019 John Wiley & Sons Ltd. Published 2019 by John Wiley & Sons Ltd.
Companion website: www.wiley.com/go/thinkinggood

> Have you got your **negative glasses** on? Are you only focusing on the negative?

> Are you **blowing things up?** Making small things bigger than they really are?

> Are you a **fortune teller** predicting what will happen?

> Are you a **mind reader** who knows what other people are thinking?

> Are you **expecting to be perfect** by setting yourself impossible standards?

> Are you **blaming yourself** for things that aren't down to you?

> Are you thinking that **positive doesn't count** and finding a way to reject any positive things that happen

> Are you **disaster thinking?** Thinking the worst possible thing that can happen?

 Challenge it

Now that you have checked for thinking traps, the next step is to look for evidence to support or challenge your thinking. Focus on the **facts** and look for things that you have overlooked, dismissed, or forgotten.

Start by finding the evidence to **support** this negative way of thinking and then look for evidence to **question** it.

> Have there been **any times when your thought is not true?** This is helpful if you are blowing things up, expecting to be perfect, or thinking that positive doesn't count?

> Is there something **important you have overlooked?** This is a helpful challenge to the negative glasses.

> What would you best friend or **someone you value say** if they heard you thinking this way? This is helpful if you are blaming yourself or looking through your negative glasses and find it hard to see another viewpoint.

> What evidence is there that this has taken place or **are you worrying that this might happen**? This is helpful if you are fortune telling or mind reading and can help you plan how you can stop your worries coming true.

> **Would it really be that terrible** if this happened? It is helpful to ask yourself this to challenge your disaster thinking and to put things in perspective.

Change it

Checking has helped you to find any thinking traps and challenging has helped you find new or overlooked information that might help you to question your thoughts. Now decide, on balance, whether there is another, more helpful way of thinking about this.

This is **not about tricking yourself** into thinking that everything is OK. This is not the case:

▶ Bad things happen.

▶ You will be criticised.

▶ People will be thoughtless and unkind.

▶ You will not always be successful.

▶ You will struggles to do some things.

But . . . there are many times we overlook things. Finding these can help you to see things in a more **balanced and helpful way**.

 Try to find a **balanced** way of thinking that acknowledges the situation but helps you to **cope** and to **feel better**.

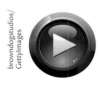

browndogstudios/ GettyImages

Sian found herself feeling very anxious in the schoolyard.

▶ She tried to **catch** the thoughts that were racing through her mind and found herself thinking that *'No one ever talks to me', 'I am stood here all on my own',* and *'Everyone thinks I am a loser'*.

▶ Sian **checked** her thoughts and found that she was in a thinking trap of **blowing things up**. She could remember plenty of times when she talked with friends at school. She was also **mind reading** by thinking that other people were judging her. When she looked around the schoolyard, they weren't interested in her and hardly anyone had noticed her on her own.

▶ Sian **challenged** this way of thinking. There was something **she had overlooked**. She was standing on her own in the schoolyard because her friends were late and hadn't come out of class yet.

▶ Sian **changed** her thoughts to something more balanced and helpful. *'My friends aren't here, so I will go and hang out with Mike.'*

This helped Sian to acknowledge the situation (haven't got my friends to talk with yet) but helped her cope (go and talk with Mike) which made her feel better (less anxious).

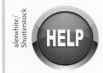

You may find this hard to start with. Don't worry, it may take time. But remember, the more you do it, the more you will be able to challenge and change the way you think.

What would someone else say?

When you are caught in a thinking trap, it can be hard to see things in a different way. If this happens, it is useful to look at things from a **different point of view**.

What would someone important to you say?

▶ What would my best friend say if they heard me thinking like this?

▶ What would someone I respect (mum/dad/teacher) say if they heard me thinking like this?

Switch places and think what you would say to someone you care about.

▶ What would I say to my best friend if I heard them thinking like this?

Sita was very tearful and feeling stressed. She was watching one of her favourite programmes on TV but was really thinking about her college work. Sita couldn't understand her maths homework and caught these thoughts tumbling through her mind.

▶ *'I've messed everything up'.*

▶ *'I'm never going to pass my exams'.*

▶ *'Even if I started work now it's too late'.*

▶ *'I'm just so stupid'.*

Sita asked herself what someone else would say.

▶ What would her best friend say?
'You know that maths isn't your strongest subject, but you have always got through the exams. You are in the top groups for everything else'.

> What would her maths teacher say?
> *'We only just started this work, and I think it will take some time before you really understand it'.*

> What would Sita say to her friends?
> *'Everyone is struggling'. 'No one knows what to do'.*

Thinking what someone else might say helped Sita to challenge her thoughts and put them in perspective. She still didn't know how to do his work, but she was able to catch and **challenge her thinking traps**.

> She was **blowing things up** – her maths homework is hard, but it is new and she is not stupid.

> She was looking through **negative glasses** – she is in the top groups for all her other subjects.

> She was **fortune telling** – predicting that it was too late to start working.

> She was **blaming herself** for being stupid – no one else can understand this work, so it is not just Sita who finds this hard.

Seeing things from a **different point of view** is sometimes easier and can help you to challenge your thoughts.

Dealing with worries

Sometimes we might find ourselves constantly worrying. No matter how hard we try to challenge our thoughts or to be mindful, the worries keep coming back and our heads feel cluttered.

We worry about many different things, and there are some worries **we can do something about** like the following:

> If you worry about getting up late, you can put an alarm on or ask someone to wake you up.

> If you worry that you will forget your homework, you can write it down on your phone or in a notebook.

> If you worry that you are gaining weight, you can cut out snacks or eat smaller portions.

There are also many worries that you can do nothing about. These are often the 'what if' types of worries like the following:

▶ *'What if the bus crashed?'*

▶ *'What if I have cancer?'*

▶ *'What if mum has an accident?'*

Why do we worry?

People think that worrying can be helpful. That it helps

▶ To solve problems and find solutions

▶ To motivate you to get things done

▶ To prepare you for all possible outcomes

▶ To prevent things going wrong or to stop bad things happening

▶ To show that you care

 In reality **worrying about things that you can do nothing about doesn't help**. It just makes you feel more anxious as you keep thinking about the negative things that could happen.

Keep worries under control

You may find that your worries start to limit what you do. If you become so worried

▶ about the school bus crashing, you might stop going on the bus.

▶ about having cancer, you might keep visiting your doctor to check that you are OK.

▶ about mum having an accident, you may want to stay with her all the time to make sure she is OK.

When this happens, your **worries have taken over**. They make you feel bad and limit what you can do.

Limit the amount of time you spend worrying. **Solve** those worries you can do something about and **accept** those that you can't solve.

Make worry time

Rather than worrying throughout the day, make a 15-minute time to worry (e.g. 5.00–5.15). During this time, you can worry about whatever you want. Chose a time that suits you but don't make it too near bed time. It might keep you awake.

Delay worry

Worries will keep tumbling through you head during the day. As they happen, write them down, but don't spend time worrying about them. You can do that later during worry time. Instead, take a few deep breaths and refocus your attention on what is going on around you.

Solve the worries you can do something about

During worry time look at your worry list. You will find that some of your worries have disappeared. For those that are still bothering you, check whether or not you can do something about them. If you can, work through your worry and work out what you can do to help. The six-step problem-solving approach can help (refer to Chapter 15).

Accept the worries you can do nothing about

You will probably have a number of 'what if' worries on your list that you can do nothing about. Learn to accept that you will worry, that some worries will be scary, and that you don't know what will happen in the future. Live for the moment. Enjoy the here and now rather than worrying about the future.

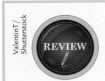

ValentinT/
Shutterstock

When you notice an unhelpful thought catch it, check it, challenge it, and change it.

Think what someone else would say if they heard your unhelpful thoughts or what you would say to a friend if you heard them thinking like this.

Limit the time you spend worrying. Solve the worries you can do something about and accept those you have no control over.

Thought checking

When you notice regular unhelpful thoughts, it can be useful to check them to see if there is another

▶ more balanced way of thinking

▶ that acknowledges the situation but

▶ makes you feel better and

▶ helps you cope

CATCH IT – What thoughts are tumbling around your head? Do they make you feel good and encourage you to do things?

CHECK IT – What thinking traps have you fallen into? Are you thinking that things are worse than they really are?

CHALLENGE IT – What is the evidence to support or challenge these thoughts? Is there something you have overlooked?

CHANGE IT – Is there another more helpful and balanced way of thinking?

What would someone else say?

When you notice unhelpful thoughts racing through your mind catch them and ask yourself what someone else would say if they heard you thinking like this?

> What thoughts are tumbling around your head?

> What would your best friend say if they heard you thinking like this?

> What would someone you respect (mum/dad/teacher) say?

> What would I say to my best friend if I heard them thinking like this?

Dealing with worries

Limit the amount of time you spend worrying by creating a daily worry time. Write down any worries that happen during the day.

> Worries that are bothering me.

During worry time, sort your worries into those you can do something about and those you can't.

> Worries I can do something about here and now. Write your plan next to each worry.

> Worries I can do nothing about.

Solve the worries you can do something about and accept those that you have no control over.

Core beliefs

Changing the way you think is not always easy. Some unhelpful thoughts seem very strong and powerful. You might be able to catch them but find it hard to challenge them or to believe that here is a different way of thinking.

The automatic thoughts that tumble around our heads are driven by some very strong ways of thinking called **core beliefs**. These develop over time and are shaped by our experiences and important events. We develop core beliefs about ourselves, how others will treat us, and what will happen.

▶ If you are constantly criticised by your parents, you might develop a core belief about yourself – *'I am rubbish'*.

▶ If you have been regularly bullied or teased, you might develop a core belief about how others treat you – *'people are out to get me'*.

▶ If you have experienced a severe traumatic event, you might develop a core belief about the future – *'Nothing will ever work out'*.

Core beliefs

Core beliefs are **very strong, rigid** ways of thinking. They are often very short sweeping statements which we apply to all situations:

▶ *'I am worthless'*.

▶ *'Others are better than me'*.

▶ *'I can't cope on my own'*.

When Sam started school, she found it very hard to make friends. The other young people left her out, called her names, teased her, and laughed at the way she dressed. This was very upsetting for Sam who spent a lot of time on

Thinking Good, Feeling Better: A Cognitive Behavioural Therapy Workbook for Adolescents and Young Adults, First Edition. Paul Stallard.
© 2019 John Wiley & Sons Ltd. Published 2019 by John Wiley & Sons Ltd.
Companion website: www.wiley.com/go/thinkinggood

her own. It is not surprising that Sam developed a very strong core belief that *'people don't like me'*.

Sam changed to a new school. The children were kinder and were keen to involve her in what they did, but Sam found it hard to recognise that the situation had changed. Her core belief was very strong, and she continued to believe that people didn't like her and so spent her free time avoiding the others.

▶ When she was with others, Sam fell into the **negative glasses** thinking trap and was always looking for signs, no matter how small, that they did not like her.

▶ Sam would over-think situations and would **blow up** small things to become evidence that she was being criticised and teased.

▶ When she was invited out, Sam would be a **fortune teller** and predict that she would be teased and laughed at.

▶ When talking, she would find herself **mind reading** and thinking that everyone thought she was boring and had nothing interesting to say.

The more Sam looked, the more evidence she found to strengthen her core belief that 'people don't like her'. Sam never questioned this and hadn't recognised that the situation had changed. Because her core belief was so powerful, she accepted it as true.

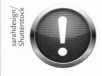

Core beliefs are **very strong and rigid** ways of thinking. They are kept strong by **thinking traps**. We **look for evidence to support** them and **dismiss anything that questions** them.

Finding core beliefs

Core beliefs are not always easy to spot. When you notice an automatic thought that

▶ **really bothers you**

▶ **produces a very strong reaction**

▶ **keeps popping up**

Write it down. Keep this going for a few days and see if there are any common patterns or themes.

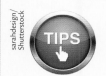

TIPS

Once you find a troubling and unhelpful thought, you can find your core belief by asking yourself '**So what does it mean**'. Keep asking yourself this question until you find the core belief which is driving your thoughts.

Alice had many worries about her mother. She didn't know why, but noticed very strong hot thoughts tumbling through her head when her mum went out in her car. Mum was a good driver and never had an accident, but Alice couldn't stop worrying. Alice asked herself the **so what does it mean** question to find the core belief that was driving her thoughts.

Mum goes out in the car

⬇

'Oh no, does mum need to go out in the car'

⬇

So what does it mean … if mum goes out in her car?

⬇

'Mum might have an accident'

⬇

So what does it mean… if mum has an accident?

⬇

'Mum might be badly hurt'

⬇

So what does it mean … if mum is badly hurt?

⬇

'Mum might end up in hospital'

⬇

So what does it mean … if mum ends up in hospital?

⬇

'No one would be there to look after me'

⬇

So what does it mean … if there is no one to look after you?

⬇

'I can't cope'

This helped Alice to understand that her worries were not about mum driving her car. She knew mum was a safe driver. Her real fear was about having to cope on her own if anything bad happened to her mum.

Alice's core belief that she 'can't cope' made her feel anxious. This helped Alice to understand why she would avoid or put off doing things until someone was around to help.

 Joe felt really angry after he was dropped from the football team. He had lots of thoughts tumbling around his head. The more he listened to his thoughts, the angrier he became. Joe decided to find out what was causing all these thoughts.

Joe is dropped from the football team

⬇

'I'm the only one they dropped'

⬇

So what does it mean … if you are the only one dropped?

⬇

'I'm the easiest person to get rid of. It's always me first. This is so unfair'

⬇

So what does it mean … if you are always the first to be dropped?

⬇

'Nobody bothers about me'

⬇

So what does it mean … if nobody bothers about you?

⬇

'I am worthless'

Joe's core belief that *'I am worthless'* made him feel angry. He as always looking for evidence that people were picking on him or treating him unfairly. This helped Joe to understand why he was always arguing with other people and getting into trouble.

 Identifying your core beliefs can help you understand some of the common feelings you have and how you behave.

Challenging core beliefs

Core beliefs are very strong and powerful. They are very rigid, general ways of thinking where you believe that your belief **will always be true.**

> If you have a core belief that you are *'worthless'*, you will **never** be valued by anyone.

> If you have a core belief that *'others are better than you'*, then you will **never** be better than anyone else at anything you do.

> If you have a core belief that *'you can't cope'*, you will **never** be able to deal with any challenges.

 This is not true. There will be times when you are valued, can do better than some of your peers, and are able to cope with challenges. It is important to find ways to **put limits around your core beliefs**.

 Is it always true?

A useful way to put limits around our core beliefs is to look for evidence that they are **not always true**. No matter how small or unimportant it may seem, we need to find evidence to question what we believe.

If you have a belief that you are worthless, you need to find evidence where people have valued you, your ideas, strengths, or skills.

> Notice when people contact you, ask for your advice, or spend time with you. Why would they do this if you were worthless?

If you have a belief that other people are better than you, look for evidence where you have been successful.

> Notice when you are not last or bottom of the class. This shows that there are times when you are more successful than others.

If you have a belief that you can't cope, look for evidence where you have been able to handle a challenge.

> Notice when you have been able to solve a problem. It may be hard, but there will be times when you are able to cope.

Put limits around your core beliefs by looking for evidence, no matter how small, that they are **not always true**.

If it doesn't work?

Changing core beliefs takes time. You may find evidence that you beliefs are not always true, but you may still find it hard to believe what you have found. Because they are so strong and powerful, you may find yourself dismissing or rejecting your evidence.

If this happens, it can be useful **to talk with someone**. Talk with a close friend or someone you respect and find out whether they see things the same way as you. Another person may help to challenge your view. They might provide new information which you have overlooked or rejected or highlight the importance of things that you find difficult to see or believe.

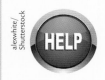

alewhite / Shutterstock

If you find it hard to challenge your core beliefs and find evidence that they are not always true, talk to someone. They might see things differently to you.

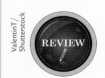

ValentinT / Shutterstock

Core beliefs are strong, rigid, powerful ways of thinking.

They are kept strong by our thinking traps. We look for evidence to support them and dismiss anything that questions them.

You can find your core beliefs by asking 'So what does this mean'.

Put limits around your core beliefs by finding evidence that they are not always true.

So what does it mean?

When you notice a thought that really bothers you or keeps popping up try asking yourself **SO WHAT** to find the belief that is driving it

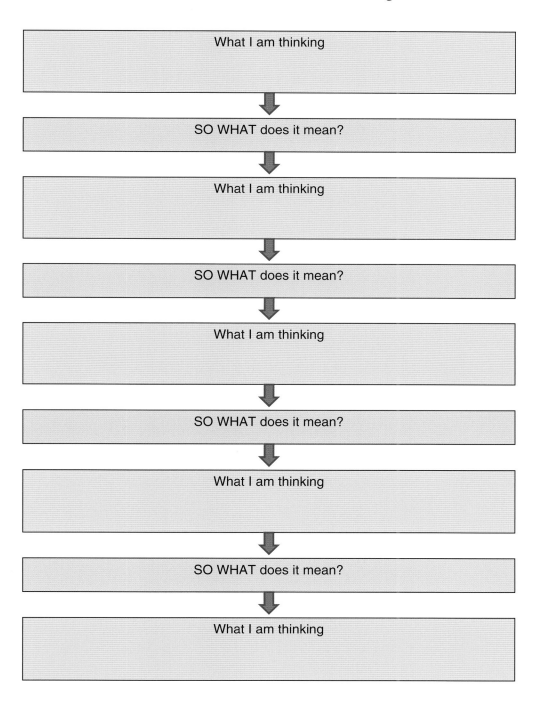

What I am thinking

SO WHAT does it mean?

What I am thinking

SO WHAT does it mean?

What I am thinking

SO WHAT does it mean?

What I am thinking

SO WHAT does it mean?

What I am thinking

Is it always true?

Write down your core belief and look for any evidence, no matter how small, that it is not always true.

My Core Belief

Evidence that this belief is not ALWAYS true.

My beliefs

To discover some of your beliefs, choose a number between 1 and 10 to show how much you believe each of the statements below

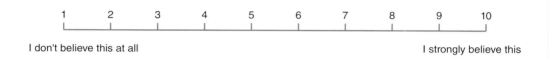

1   2   3   4   5   6   7   8   9   10

I don't believe this at all   I strongly believe this

	Belief rating
It is important to be better than others at everything I do.	
Other people are better than me.	
No one loves or cares about me.	
It is important that my parents/carers are involved in everything I do.	
I am not responsible for what I do or say.	
I am a failure.	
I am more important/special than others.	
People will be cross or upset if I say the things I really want to say.	
I must not show my feelings to others.	
It is more important to put other people's wishes and ideas before my own.	
Others are out to get or hurt me.	
No one understands me.	
People I love will never be there for me.	
I need other people to help me get by.	
Bad things happen to me.	

Understand how you feel

Each day you will notice a number of different feelings. You may **feel**

▷ **sad** when someone says something unkind

▷ **happy** talking with your friends

▷ **angry** if you are criticised

▷ **anxious** when you have to do something new

▷ **relaxed** listening to music

Your feelings will change throughout the day. You may not always notice how you feel. Your feelings might be very weak and may not last very long. At other times, they might be very strong. They may seem to last a long time and **interfere with what you do**.

▷ If you feel **sad**, it can be **hard to motivate** yourself to do things.

▷ If you feel **angry**, it can be **hard to solve** problems.

▷ If you feel **anxious**, you **may avoid** things that worry you.

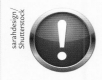

When your feelings take over, you need to regain control of your life and learn how you can help yourself to feel better.

Body signals

We are not always very good at identifying our feelings or may wrap them up together under one label 'I feel rubbish'.

Thinking Good, Feeling Better: A Cognitive Behavioural Therapy Workbook for Adolescents and Young Adults, First Edition. Paul Stallard.
© 2019 John Wiley & Sons Ltd. Published 2019 by John Wiley & Sons Ltd.
Companion website: www.wiley.com/go/thinkinggood

To understand more about how you feel, it is helpful to identify the **body signals** that tell you when you feel sad, anxious, or angry.

▶ When you feel **sad**, you might notice body signals like crying, feeling tired, becoming short-tempered, and finding it hard to concentrate. You might notice changes in your appetite or sleeping, become quiet or spend more time on your own.

▶ When you feel **anxious**, you might notice body signals like a racing heart, rapid breathing, and feeling hot and sweaty. You may shake, put off doing things, or want others to be with you.

▶ When you feel **angry**, you might notice body signals like feeling hot, going red, clenching your fists, or a racing heart. You may shout, swear, argue, or stamp around.

Different **emotions can share** the same body signals. For example

▶ your heart might race fast if you are angry or anxious

▶ you may become quiet and withdrawn if you are anxious or sad

▶ you may be irritable and shout if you are sad or angry

To get better at identifying your different feelings, try to identify **all your body signals** connected with each feeling.

Feelings

Although your feelings may seem fairly random, they don't just suddenly happen. There is often a reason.

If you check what happens carefully, you will probably find that your feelings are connected with **what you do**.

▶ You may feel, happy at home, sad at work, and worried when you go somewhere new.

▶ You may feel relaxed watching TV, angry doing your homework, and anxious when you go swimming.

- You may feel sad when you are with your dad, happy with your best friend, and angry with your brother.

Feelings are also connected with the **way you think**. Some ways of thinking are helpful and make us feel good and others are unhelpful and make us feel unpleasant.

- If you think, *'I played well in that game'*, or *'Look good in these clothes'*, you will probably feel happy.

- If you think *'I played terribly today'*, or *'I look terrible in these clothes'*, you will probably feel sad or angry.

Feelings are connected with **what you do** and **how you think**.

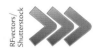

How do your feelings change?

To find out how your feelings change throughout the day, it can be useful to keep a feeling diary. You can do this in two ways:

- When you **notice a strong feeling** write down how you felt, what you were doing, who was there, and what you were thinking.

- You could also **check in with your feelings** each day. Check how you feel in the morning, afternoon, and evening. Write down the feeling you discovered, what you were doing, who was there, and any thoughts you catch.

At the end of the week, look at your diary and find out whether there are any patterns.

- What are the feelings you notice most often?

- Are there any places that seem to trigger these feelings?

- Do they happen with particular people – crowds, friends, and family?

- Are there any particular thoughts associated with your feelings?

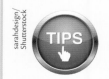

Keep a diary to find out what places, people, and thoughts are connected to your feelings.

Why me?

When feelings persist and become very strong, you might become depressed or have an anxiety problem. These are common with about one in five young people suffering with anxiety or depression before the age of 18.

Feeling depressed or anxious is horrible, so **don't beat yourself up** for feeling like this. You **didn't choose to feel like this**. It just happened. There often isn't one reason why people become anxious or depressed. It is a mix of different things including your **genes**, what happens in your **life**, and **you**.

Genes

Anxiety and depression run in families. If one of your parents is depressed or anxious, you could inherit a gene that increases the risk of you developing anxiety or depression. This is a small risk, and even if your parents were anxious or depressed, it does not automatically mean that you will become depressed or anxious.

Life

Anxiety and depression can be triggered by life events. Someone close to you may die; you may have been involved in a trauma, been bullied, or be unwell; your mum and dad may have had problems getting on or you may have had lots of house or school moves. We cope well with many changes, but sometimes these can become too much and make us feel anxious or depressed.

You

Some people are pessimistic, worry about what will happen and always look on the gloomy side of life. This way of thinking will make you feel worried and sad and can drag you down so that you become anxious or depressed.

You may not know why you became depressed or anxious. The **good news** is that it doesn't always matter. You can **help yourself to get better** by changing your approach to life.

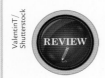

ValentinT/Shutterstock

We can become better at identifying our feelings by understanding our body signals.

Feelings don't just randomly happen. They are often associated with what we do and how we think.

A diary can help you find out more about your feelings. Understanding your feelings can help you learn to control them, so that you feel better.

Feeling down

What signals do you notice when you feel sad, upset, or down?

▶ Feel tired

▶ Go off your food

▶ Comfort eat

▶ Cry

▶ Feel irritable and short-tempered

▶ Can't be bothered to do things

▶ Have difficulty falling asleep

▶ Wake up early in the morning

▶ Can't concentrate

▶ Go out less

▶ Stop doing things that you like or enjoy

▶ Have thoughts about wanting to hurt yourself

Any other signals you notice?

Feeling anxious

What signals do you notice when you feel scared, frightened, or anxious?

▶ Racing heart

▶ Short of breath

▶ Hot or sweaty

▶ Red in the face

▶ Shake

▶ Butterflies in tummy or feeling sick

▶ Dry mouth

▶ Mind goes blank

▶ Headache

▶ Want to go to the toilet

▶ Light-headed or feel faint

Any other signals you notice?

Feeling angry

What signals do you notice when you feel cross, angry, or uptight?

▶ Feel hot, go red in the face

▶ Argue

▶ Raise your voice/shout

▶ Swear or abuse people

▶ Clench your fists

▶ Grind you teeth

▶ Feel tense

▶ Throw things

▶ Slam doors

▶ Lash out, hit, kick

▶ Stamp around

Any other signals you notice?

Do others feel like me?

It often feels as if we are the only one who ever becomes down in their mood or anxious. Check this out to see how common this is?

Search on the Internet to see if you can find answers to these questions?

How many young people suffer with depression?

How many young people suffer with anxiety?

Find three famous people who have suffered with depression.

Find three famous people who have suffered with anxiety.

What did they do to overcome their problems?

Feeling diary

Feelings don't just randomly happen, so keep a diary to help you understand what triggers your feelings. Whenever you notice a strong feeling write down

▶ how you felt

▶ what you were doing and who was there

▶ what you were thinking

Day and time	How you felt	What were you doing and who was there	What were you thinking

Are your feelings connected to what you do or how you think?

Mood monitoring

Our feelings vary throughout the day. Mood monitoring will help you to understand how your feelings change, and the times that are most difficult for you.

For each part of the day, choose the feeling that you have noticed most and choose a number between 1 and 10 to show strong it has been.

1 = Very weak to 10 = Very strong

	Woke up	Mid-morning	Lunch	After school	Tea time	Bed
Monday						
Tuesday						
Wednesday						
Thursday						
Friday						
Saturday						
Sunday						

Are there any days or times which are particularly difficult?

Control your feelings

Feelings can become very strong and hard to control. They may take over and stop you from doing the things you would really like to do.

▶ You may **want** to go out, but because you **feel so unhappy**, you can't be bothered.

▶ You may **want** to be with your friends, but because you **feel so angry**, you end up arguing, and your friends don't invite you out anymore.

▶ You may **want** to call a friend, but because **you feel so anxious**, you are unable to do so.

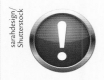

When your feelings take over you might **put things off, avoid** things that are challenging, or **stop doing** the things you used to enjoy. You end up doing less and less and spend more time at home on our own.

You don't have to let your feelings control what you do. Try some of these ideas, and see if they can help you to manage your emotions. Keep an open mind and find out what methods work for you.

Relaxation exercises

Many famous celebrities, athletes, and musicians use relaxation exercises to help them prepare for challenges. Relaxation involves tensing each of the major muscle groups in your body and then releasing the tension. **Tensing the muscles helps them to relax**.

There are a number of audio guides that will take your though the process of tensing and relaxing your muscles. If you don't have one, you can follow the instructions below.

Thinking Good, Feeling Better: A Cognitive Behavioural Therapy Workbook for Adolescents and Young Adults, First Edition. Paul Stallard.
© 2019 John Wiley & Sons Ltd. Published 2019 by John Wiley & Sons Ltd.
Companion website: www.wiley.com/go/thinkinggood

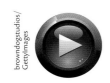

Choose a time when you won't be interrupted. Find a quiet, warm place and turn your phone off. Lie down or sit comfortably. You may want to shut your eyes, but if you want to keep them open that's fine.

▶ Tense each muscle group twice. Tense it enough so that it feels tight, but don't hurt yourself.

▶ Start by taking five deep breaths. Slowly breathe in through your nose and out through your mouth.

▶ Now turn your attention to your feet and curl up your toes. Scrunch them up, count to 5 and release them. **Notice the difference between tension and relaxation**. Tense them again.

▶ Move your attention to your legs and tense your calves by pointing your toes towards your knees. Count to 5, release the tension and notice the difference between tension and relaxation.

▶ Tense your thighs by pushing the back of your legs against the chair or bed.

▶ Move to your stomach and tense this by sucking in your stomach and pushing your belly button towards your spine.

▶ Focus on your arms and hands and tense them by making a tight fist and curling your arms up towards your shoulders.

▶ Now tense your back by arching your spine and pushing your shoulder blades together. Count to 5, relax and notice the difference between tension and relaxation.

▶ Focus on your neck and shoulders and push your shoulders up towards your ears.

▶ Shift your attention to your face and tense your chin and jaw by clenching your teeth and pushing your chin down towards your chest.

▶ Finally, tense the rest of the muscles in your face by closing your eyes and pressing your lips together tightly and screw up you face.

▶ As you release each muscle notice the tension fade away.

▶ Return your attention to your breathing and enjoy this relaxed feeling for a few minutes.

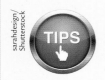

Try building relaxation exercises into your daily routine. If you did this before bed, it might help you to sleep better.

Quick relaxation

There may be times when you don't have time to tense and relax each of your muscles. A quicker way of doing this is to **tense each of the major muscle groups together**.

Tense your muscles, hold them for five seconds, and as you breathe out let them go and notice the tension fade away. Repeat this and enjoy that nice calm feeling for a couple of minutes.

▶ *Arms and hands*: Clench your fists and push your arms towards your shoulders.

▶ *Legs and feet*: Push your toes towards your knees, gently raise your legs, and stretch them out in front of you.

▶ *Stomach*: Suck your tummy in.

▶ *Shoulders and neck*: Push your shoulders up towards your ears and pull your shoulders blades together.

▶ *Face*: Screw up your face, squeeze your eyes and jaw tightly, and push your lips together.

▶ The more you practice the easier you will find this.

Make a regular time each day to relax. Making it part of your daily routine will remind you to practice.

Physical activity

A natural way of tensing and relaxing your muscles is through physical activity. Activity can also improve your mood. **When you exercise, your brain produces chemicals which make you feel good**.

You can do as little or as much physical activity as you want. The idea is to do enough to release the tension in your body. Think about the exercise you enjoy. It could be anything like

▶ swimming

▶ tennis

- football

- basketball

- dance

- a workout

- cycling

- running

- jogging

- walking

- cleaning your room

 TIPS   If you are feeling stressed, try doing some form of physical activity to help you relax.

 ## 4-5-6 breathing

When people become anxious, they often notice that their breathing changes. They start to breathe in short, shallow, fast breaths. This is part of a normal reaction designed to keep you safe called the 'fight or flight response'. When this happens, you breathe in more oxygen to give your body the fuel, it needs to deal with the threat that is making you anxious – run away or fight it off. **Controlling your breathing can help you relax and regain control**.

 This is a quick way to regain control of your breathing and to calm down. It is very simple and can be used anywhere. People will probably not even notice what you are doing.

- Breath in slowly through your mouth to the count of 4

- Hold the breath to the count of 5

- Slowly breathe out through your mouth to the count of 6

- Repeat three times.

When you notice your breathing change or you are starting to feel stressed try 4-5-6 breathing. It is very quick, so try and practice two or three times each day.

Calming images

We can use our **imagination to create a special calming place** which can help us to feel relaxed, peaceful, and happy.

You need to practice creating an image of your special place. When you feel stressed, you can go there in your mind to relax and unwind.

▶ Your calming place should be somewhere that feels very special to you. It could be somewhere that you have been which has good memoires or an imaginary place like floating in space.

▶ To help you create a good image find a photograph or draw a picture of your calming place.

▶ Practice creating this image in your mind and try to make it as real as possible by describing:

- **what you see** – the colours of the sky and sand and the shapes of the rocks
- **what you hear** – the sound of waves crashing on the beach and the noise of seagulls shrieking
- **what you feel** – the wind blowing through your hair and the sun warming your face
- **what you smell** – the smell of sun screen and the smoky BBQ
- **what you taste** – the salty water in your mouth

▶ Practice imaging your calming place. If you notice yourself feeling anxious or stressed, then create your calming image and imagine you are there.

When you feel uptight, try to create your relaxing place and go there in your mind to relax and calm down.

Mind games

You may find that you notice your thoughts and body signals more when you get anxious or feel down. The more you focus on them, the worse they get.

Mind games are a **quick and easy way of distracting yourself** from unhelpful thoughts and unpleasant feelings. They help you to focus on the things that are going on around you rather than your internal thoughts and body signals. You can do this in many ways such as

▶ Naming an animal with each letter of the alphabet

▶ Counting backwards from 147 in eights

▶ Spelling the names of family or friends backwards

▶ Using the letters from car number plates to make words

Mind games can help you get some short-term relief. The mind game needs to be hard enough to make you think and try to do it as quickly as you can.

Change the feeling

Often, we notice how we feel, but don't do anything to make ourselves feel better. It seems as if our feelings are in charge and control us. This isn't the case. There are many things we can do to help ourselves feel better.

If you notice an unpleasant feeling, don't just live with it, change it. You can do this by doing something that makes you feel good.

▶ If you are **feeling tense** try and do something that **helps you relax**. It could be having a long bath, drawing, having a massage, listening to your favourite music, or reading a book.

▶ If you are **feeling unhappy**, try and do something that helps **you feel good**. It could be watching your favourite comedy, painting your nails, baking a cake, or playing with a pet.

▶ If you are **feeling angry** try and do something that helps **you calm down**. It could be going on the Internet, hitting a cushion or punch bag, watching TV, popping bubble wrap, or going for a walk.

It is useful to make a list of the things that can help you to change the way you feel. This is a helpful way of reminding yourself what might help when you feel unhappy, angry or anxious.

Soothe yourself

Sometimes we might blame ourselves or feel guilty about things and think that we deserve to feel bad. No one deserves to feel bad, so you need to be kinder to yourself. Look after yourself and **find ways to soothe and comfort yourself**.

One way you can soothe yourself is by stimulating your senses with things you find pleasurable. Really concentrate on what you are doing and don't let your mind wander. Pretend it is the first time you have ever smelt, touched, tasted, seen, or heard these things. Find what works for you and what stimulates your senses:

- **Smell** – your favourite perfume, soap, fresh coffee, or scented candle
- **Touch** – a smooth stone, soft toy, silky fabric, or take a warm bath
- **Taste** – a chewy sweet, soft marshmallow, strong mint, refreshing apple, or tangy orange
- **Sight** – pictures or quotes that make you smile, watching a fish tank, or clouds drifting in the sky
- **Hearing** – your favourite music, birds singing, sound of the trees blowing in the wind

Once you have identified the things you find soothing, try and put them together. You now have a soothing kit ready to be used whenever you need it.

Talk to someone

Whilst other people can often be the cause of our distress and unhappiness, they can also help us to feel better.

If you are feeling down or anxious, don't sit on your own. If you do, you will probably find yourself rehearsing what has happened or worrying about what will happen. Instead of this decide

▶ **Who could you talk with?** Who makes you feel good?

▶ **What do you want to tell them?** Do you want to share how you are feeling or to talk about other things?

▶ **What do you want them to do?** Do you need someone to listen to you, give you a hug, or help to sort out a problem? You need to tell them what you want.

▶ **How will you contact them?** You can arrange to meet them, telephone, text, email, or use social media.

▶ **When will you contact them?** As soon as possible so that you can start to feel better.

Get a list of 'feel good' people who you can contact when you are feeling down or unhappy.

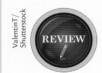

When you feel unpleasant, don't just live with it. Do something to make yourself feel better.

Develop your own toolbox to manage your emotions.

These methods won't always work, but the more you practice, the more help they will be.

Relaxing diary

When you notice a strong unpleasant feeling try doing some relaxation exercises. Rate the strength of your feeling from 1 to 100 before and after you have used your relaxation exercises.

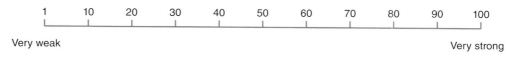

| 1 | 10 | 20 | 30 | 40 | 50 | 60 | 70 | 80 | 90 | 100 |

Very weak   Very strong

Day and time	How did you feel before 1–100	What did you do to change the feeling	How did you feel after 1–100

Activities that help me feel better

Physical activity can help you to feel better. When you feel stressed, unhappy, or angry, try a physical activity to see if it helps. What activities might help you?

> What sports do you enjoy? Swimming, tennis, football, or basketball?

> What physical activities you enjoy? Dance, workout, cycle, run, or jog?

> Are there other physical things you enjoy? Walking, mowing the lawn, or shopping?

My calming place

When you feel anxious or uptight, try to create a calming place in your mind which you can use to help you calm down. This can be a real place or somewhere you have created in your dreams.

▶ Draw or find a picture of your calming place

▶ Choose a quiet time when you will not be disturbed and turn off your phone

▶ Shut your eyes and create a picture of your calming place

▶ Make it as detailed as possible

▶ Explore the colours, shapes, and sizes

▶ Listen for any sounds

▶ Notice any smells

▶ Enjoy any tastes

▶ Notice any pleasant feelings like the sun warming your face

▶ Notice how relaxed you have become

Enjoy this feeling and return to your calming place whenever you want.

The more you practice, the easier it will be to create you calming place and the quicker you will become calm.

Change the feeling

When you feel unpleasant, try to change the feeling by doing something you enjoy and makes you feel good. What makes you feel good?

What makes you feel relaxed? A long bath, drawing, listening to your favourite music, or reading a book?

What makes you feel happy? Watching your favourite comedy, painting your nails, baking a cake, or playing with a pet?

What makes you feel calm? Surfing the Internet, playing an instrument, watching TV, or going for a walk?

Soothing toolbox

Develop a soothing toolbox of things that please each of your senses. Once you have identified what you enjoy put them together so that they are ready when you need them.

What **SMELLS** do you enjoy? Perfume, soap, spice, coffee, or scented candle?

What **TOUCH** do you enjoy? Smooth stone, soft toy, silky fabric, or warm bath?

What **TASTE** do you enjoy? Chewy sweet, strong mint, refreshing apple, or tangy orange?

What **SIGHTS** do you enjoy? Pictures or quotes, fish tank, or clouds?

What **SOUNDS** do you enjoy? Music, birds, or tress blowing in the wind?

Talk to someone

There are many things you can do to help yourself feel better, but sometimes it might be helpful to talk with someone else.

Who could you talk with?

What do you want to tell them?

What do you want them to do?

How will you contact them?

When will you do it?

Problem-solving

Every day we face a number of challenges where we have to make decisions about what we are going to do.

▶ If you are teased, you could walk away **OR** fight back.

▶ If your tutor asks you to be quiet, you could do as they say **OR** carry on talking.

▶ If your friend tells you a secret, you could keep it private **OR** share it with someone else.

▶ If your parents ask you to help at home, you could do it **OR** put it off.

Some decisions are quite **easy** to make. There may be **fewer choices** and it is very **clear** what will happen.

▶ You either stop talking or continue. If you continue, your tutor may ask you to leave the lesson.

▶ You either help at home, or you don't. If you don't, your parents may stop your allowance.

Other decisions are **more complicated**. There may **not be one answer**.

▶ If you ignore the teasing, it may get worse, but if you report it, the bullies may be angry and threaten you.

▶ If you share the secret, you may keep your friend safe, but you may fall out, and they may never trust you again.

Whatever you choose, your decision will have **consequences** for **you** and the **others** involved.

▶ Reporting the teasing may stop it and make you feel happier. The bullies might get into trouble and excluded from school.

Thinking Good, Feeling Better: A Cognitive Behavioural Therapy Workbook for Adolescents and Young Adults, First Edition.
Paul Stallard.
© 2019 John Wiley & Sons Ltd. Published 2019 by John Wiley & Sons Ltd.
Companion website: www.wiley.com/go/thinkinggood

There may also be different consequences in the **short** and **long** term.

▶ If you share the secret, your friend may stop talking to you. Over time they may realise that you were being helpful and you may become friends again.

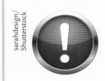

We need to think through our decisions so that we are clear about the consequences.

Why do problems happen?

We don't set out to create problems. It is the decisions we make that create problems, and this can happen in different ways.

We put decisions off.
Making decisions can be hard. We might chose to put off or ignore our problems and hope they go away. Unfortunately, challenges and hassles don't go away. They keep coming and may build up so that you feel totally overwhelmed.

We rush into decisions.
We may make poor decisions because we don't think things through. You may retaliate and hit the person who is teasing you. As you walk away, you may feel good, but in the longer term, you may be excluded from school.

Feelings take over.
Our emotions may get in the way and stop us from thinking through the consequences. When your teacher asks you to be quiet, you may think that your teacher is picking on you. You may become angry, shout, and swear and get into even more trouble as your angry feelings take over.

There is no easy decision.
Decisions can be very complicated. The secret your friend has shared may be about them choosing to do something risky. You may be concerned for their safety and so share their secret with someone else, but your friend may be angry with you.

Always done it this way.
We become fixed in our ideas and behave in the same way. This is OK as long as what we do is successful. Problems happen when we keep making the same mistakes time and time again.

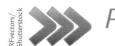

Problem-solving

Problem-solving is a useful way of helping us decide how to deal with challenges and problems and involves six steps:

- **Stop. What decision do you need to make?**

- **What are your choices?**

- **What are the consequences of your choices?**

- **On balance, what will you chose to do?**

- **Do it.**

- **Did it work?**

Stop. What decision do you need to make?

The first step is to define your problem and the decisions you need to make. Be specific. It may feel that 'life' and 'everything' is a challenge, but try and define clearly what you need to do. This stops you rushing in and allows any strong emotions to pass so that you are calm and able to think.

What are your choices?

The next step is to explore all the different decisions you could make. This will help you to think about different ways of doing things so that you don't make the same old mistakes.

A useful way of creating ideas is to keep asking yourself a simple question. I could do . . . ..OR . . . . .. OR . . . . ..OR . . . ? Try to come up with as many ideas as possible.

What are the consequences?

Check the consequences of each idea. Think about the immediate and longer-term consequences. Think about the consequences for you and for others who might be involved. This will help you think through complicated decisions where there isn't an easy decision.

On balance what will you do?

Now that you have worked out the consequences of each decision, the next step is to decide what you will do. On balance, what do you think is the best decision you could make?

Did it work?

This final step is important. Ask yourself whether you would make this decision again. Was it a good decision, and if not, what would you differently.

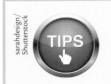

Don't rush in or delay making decisions. Use these six steps to help you make the best decisions to solve your problems.

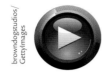

Robbie was always arguing with his parents. Robbie liked to play his music really loud, but his parents would complain and tell him to turn it down. This had been going on for weeks with Robbie ignoring his parents. Yesterday, the argument was really bad with Robbie and his dad almost having a fight. Robbie didn't want this to happen and so decided he needed to do something different.

Stop. What decision do you need to make?

Robbie didn't want to get into a fight with his dad. This was more likely to happen if he played his music loud. Robbie didn't want to stop listening to his music, so he had to work out how he could listen to his music without getting into arguments.

What are your choices?

Robbie was still feeling quite angry, and to start with, he could only think of one option. He would play has music at the same volume, but would lock his door so his dad couldn't get in. He knew this would only make things worse, but he felt angry. Robbie pushed himself to come up with other options:

▶ Play my music loud, but lock the door so dad can't get in
OR

▶ Turn the volume down
OR

▶ Play my music loud when my parents are out, but turn it down when they are at home
OR

▶ Buy some headphones

What are the consequences of your choices?

▶ If Robbie played his music loud and locked the door, he would enjoy his music and feel good. But Robbie would also feel worried. He knew that he would be winding his dad up, and there was a chance they could end up fighting. Even if they didn't fight, he wondered whether his parents would take away his sound system, and Robbie was clear that he didn't want that to happen.

▶ If Robbie turned his music down, his parents would be happier, but Robbie wouldn't. He didn't think his music would sound so good.

► If Robbie played his music loud when they were out, and quieter when they were at home, there would be less arguments. The more Robbie thought about this, he realised that his parents were at home most of the time he was at home. He would have few chances to play his music loud.

► If Robbie got some headphones his parents would be happy and Robbie could play his music as loud as he liked whenever he wanted it. But he didn't have any money to buy any headphones.

On balance, what will you chose to do?
After thinking it through, Robbie decided that if he kept playing his music loud, he would keep getting into arguments with his parents. Playing it quietly wouldn't work for Robbie, but having some headphones meant that he could still enjoy his music. It was a win–win solution, and everyone would be happy.

Do it.
Robbie decided to talk with his parents. Before he talked, he made sure, he was calm so that he didn't end up in another argument.

Robbie said that things got out of hand last night, and he didn't want this to happen again. He told them about the idea of headphones and asked if they could buy him some. His dad was still feeling angry and asked why he should spend money on Robbie when he just ignored everything they asked him to do.

Robbie thought this might happen and so suggested a compromise. He offered to keep his music quiet for the next two weeks, and in return asked if his parents could loan him the money for the headphones.

Did it work?
Robbie didn't play his music that night. The next day, he asked again, and his parents agreed to lend him the money if his music was quiet for the next two weeks.

Robbie managed this and got his headphones. More importantly, Robbie and his dad had fewer arguments and started to get on better.

Break it down

There are times when our **problems and challenges seem too big**. We know what we need to do, but our challenge feels too hard to successfully tackle in one go.

At these times, it is useful to **break your challenge into smaller steps**. If you wanted to run a marathon, you wouldn't try and run one straight away. You would start by running shorter distances. These would increase over time until you were able to run the marathon.

Break your challenges into **smaller steps**. Tackling one step at a time will be easier, and it will help you to be successful.

To break your challenge down:

▶ Write at the top of a page, **what you would like to do** (your goal) and at the bottom of the page, where you are now.

▶ Think about some of **the steps you can take** that will move you from where you are now towards achieving your goal. Write the steps on post-it notes or pieces of paper.

▶ The number of steps depends on you. There can be as many or as few as you need but make sure that the **steps aren't too big**.

▶ Give each step a **difficulty rating** from 1 (not at all difficult) to 10 (really hard).

▶ Finally, arrange the **steps in order of difficulty**. Start at the bottom, and decide what would be the first, the easiest step to take and then put the other steps in order.

Barry needed to go for an interview before he could start college. He had never had an interview or been to college and was unsure how he would get there or find his way around. It felt too much for Barry, and he had not turned up for the last two interviews. He had one last chance if he wanted to go to college next term. Barry decided to break his problem into smaller steps. Breaking the task into small steps felt more manageable for Barry.

Steps	Task	Difficulty 1–10
Step 6	My goal – Go for interview at college	9.5
Step 5	Arrange a mock interview with my teacher	7
Step 4	Go with my teacher, meet the head of studies, and look around	5
Step 3	Ask my teacher to arrange a meeting with college	4
Step 2	Go on the bus to college and check how long it takes	2.5
Step 1	Find out the times of the buses that go to college	1
Where I am	Never been to college.	

If challenges feel too big, try breaking them down into smaller steps.

Don't put off or rush into decisions. Use a problem-solving approach to help you decide what to do.

Step 1: What decision do you need to make?

Step 2: What are your choices?

Step 3: What are the consequences of your choices?

Step 4: On balance, what will you chose to do?

Step 5: Do it.

Step 6: Did it work?

If challenges feel too big, break them down into smaller steps. This will help you to be successful.

Problem-solving

If you have to make a big or a difficult decision, try to use these six steps to help you decide what you will do.

STOP. WHAT DECISION DO YOU NEED TO MAKE?

WHAT ARE YOUR CHOICES?

1.   OR
2.   OR
3.   OR
4.   OR
5.   OR

WHAT ARE THE CONSEQUENCES? For you and others in the short and long term

1.
2.
3.
4.
5.

ON BALANCE WHAT WILL YOU DO?

DID IT WORK? What would you do differently next time?

Break it down

If you challenge feels too difficult, break it down into smaller steps. Use as many steps as you need. Rate each step 1(not all difficult) to 10 (very difficult). Start with the easiest step and work towards your goal.

What I want to do (my goal)	Difficulty
Step 8	
Step 7	
Step 6	
Step 5	
Step 4	
Step 3	
Step 2	
Step 1	
Where I am now	

Check it out

Thoughts are constantly tumbling around in our heads. We hear them so often that we simply accept them as true and rarely stop to question or challenge them.

We can explore our thoughts by **thought checking** where we

▶ **Catch** the thoughts that make us feel unpleasant or talk us out of doing things.

▶ **Check** if we are caught in a thinking trap. Are we making things out to be worse than they really are?

▶ **Challenge** what we are thinking by looking for evidence that supports and questions our thoughts. Is there something positive we have overlooked?

▶ **Change** to a more balanced way of thinking which makes us feel better and helps us to be successful.

Thought checking can be helpful, but sometimes our thoughts are very strong. We may find new information that challenge our ways of thinking, but still dismiss this as unimportant.

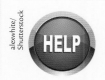

alexwhite/
Shutterstock

If you find it hard to challenge your thoughts **check out** your beliefs and predictions. Be a scientist, do an experiment, and see what actually happens.

Thinking Good, Feeling Better: A Cognitive Behavioural Therapy Workbook for Adolescents and Young Adults, First Edition.
Paul Stallard.
© 2019 John Wiley & Sons Ltd. Published 2019 by John Wiley & Sons Ltd.
Companion website: www.wiley.com/go/thinkinggood

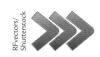

Experiments

Experiments can help us **test** whether our predictions and thoughts are **always** right and to **discover** what might happen if we did things **differently**.

Rather than talking and reasoning with ourselves, we can do an experiment to check out **exactly what happens**.

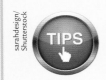

Experiments can help to put some limits around our thoughts and help us discover new information that might give us a different way of understanding the things that happen.

There are six steps to setting up an experiment.

Step 1: What thought or prediction do you want to test?

Find the negative beliefs or predictions you hear most often, that make you feel really unpleasant, or stop you from doing things. These could be things like

▶ *'No one ever invites me to do things'.*

▶ *'I am a failure'.*

Once you have chosen your thought write down a number from 1 (I don't believe this at all) to 100 (I very strongly believe this) to show much you believe it.

Step 2: What experiment could you do to test this thought?

Think of an experiment you could do to check out whether your thoughts or predictions always come true.

▶ If you thought *'No one ever calls me'*, you could keep a diary of any texts, emails, phone calls, Facebook hits, or invitations for the next seven days.

▶ If you thought you are *'a failure'*, you could keep a diary of your next five school grades.

Make sure that you will be safe during your experiment and decide when you will do it.

▶ If your phone or computer isn't working, it will not be a good time to check if people call you.

▶ If you have lots of college work for one subject, it may be better to wait until you have some different subjects to do.

Step 3: What do you think will happen?

Write down what you think will happen if your thoughts were true. This is your prediction or your assumption.

▶ If you think that *'No one ever calls'*, you might predict that you will have no text, email, phone calls, Facebook hits, or invitations over the next seven days.

▶ If you think you are *'a failure'*, you might expect that your next five grades for your college work will be D or lower.

Step 4: What happened?

Carry out your experiment and write down **exactly what happened**. This is really important. Don't dismiss or overlook anything.

Step 5: What have you found out?

Compare your prediction (Step 3) with what actually happened (Step 4). For example

▶ You predicted no messages but had three texts from your friend Jo

▶ You predicted D grades or lower. You failed two pieces of work and got two D grades, but you also got a B grade in your sport assessment.

So what have you discovered from this experiment?

▶ Are you predicting that things **will be worse than they really are**?

▶ Are you thoughts always right or **are things sometimes different?**

▶ Is there a different way of thinking which **explains** what actually happened?

    ▶ 'I don't get many calls, but Jo keeps in touch'.
    ▶ 'I struggle with my lessons, but I do well with sport'.

Step 6: Has this changed your belief or prediction?

After your experiment, chose a number from 1 to 100 to show how much you now believe the thought or prediction you wrote at Step 1. This may not have changed much because these ways of thinking are very strong and may not change very easily. You may find yourself dismissing what has happened.

▶ 'This was a good week, Jo doesn't usually text me.'

▶ 'I like football, but I am hopeless at all the other sports.'

If this happens, do another experiment and **check it out again**.

▶ Keep the diary of contacts for another two weeks.

▶ Record your next 10 college grades.

Be open-minded and curious

Whatever happens, the experiment will help you discover how things can change.

▶ You may find that no one makes contact. If this happened, you may need to become more active. Rather than waiting for someone to make contact, you could try and do things differently. Who could you contact and how could you do it?

▶ You may find that your next five college grades are bad. If that happened, you may need to talk with your tutor about the help you need to improve them or check out other parts of your life where you might be more successful.

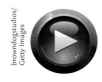

browndogstudios/
Getty Images

Mina felt very worried talking with people and often avoided social situations. She had received an invitation to a party and was worried about going. Lots of people were excited about the party and so Mina thought that she would do an experiment to check out her worries.

Step 1: What thought or prediction do you want to test?
Mina predicted that *'No one will talk with me, I will be left on my own'* if she went to the party. Mina strongly believed this, 85/100.

Step 2: What experiment could you do to test this thought?
Usually, this worry stopped Mina from going out. Today, she decided to do something different and to check out her prediction by going to the party. Mina decided she would go to the party tonight at 9.00 pm and would stay for at least 30 minutes. She was friendly with one of the girls who was going, Sophie, and decided she would say hello to her when she arrived.

Step 3: What do you think will happen?
'Sophie will say hello and then ignore me. I will stand around on my own looking stupid'.

Step 4: What happened?
Arrived at the party at 9.00 pm and found Sophie on her own. Sophie was very friendly, and we stayed together talking until I went home at 10.30 pm. I enjoyed myself.

Step 5: What have you found out?
Sophie seemed interested in talking with me. I didn't stand around on my own, and I had fun.

Step 6: Has this changed your belief or prediction?

How strongly Mina believed her original prediction had gone down to 65/100. This helped Mina to find a different way of thinking that better fitted the facts. 'I find it hard to talk with others, but people may not ignore me.'

TIPS

If you have strong ways of thinking that make you feel unhappy or stop you from doing things, **check them out**. Do an experiment and see **what actually happens**.

Surveys and searches

We often end up convinced that our understanding of the things that happen is right. At times like this, **surveys and Internet searches** can help to check whether there might be any **different explanations**.

Mike noticed that when he became worried his heart would pound loudly. Mike worried that there was something seriously wrong with him and that he would have a heart attack. His dad had a heart attack, and Mike worried that the same would happen to him. This worry kept tumbling around his head, but he never talked about it with anyone. He felt too scared.

Mike hadn't planned to do a survey, but one happened during a lesson at school when they were talking about anxiety. The teacher talked about different anxiety signals and asked how many people noticed their heart pounding loudly when they were anxious. Mike was surprised to see that other people noticed this and was relieved that he was not the only one. This also gave Mike a different understanding of what a pounding heart might mean – he was anxious and wasn't going to have a heart attack.

Jess had odd random thoughts which popped into his head. These thoughts were spooky and often were about saying or doing unkind things to others. Jess was worried that he was going mad and that he would actually do these things.

Jess decided that he would ask his friends whether they had spooky thoughts. He was embarrassed and ashamed by some of his thoughts and so couldn't talk directly to his friends. Instead, Jess decided to post a message saying he had heard a story about someone who had random spooky thoughts and wondered if anyone else ever had these. Jess was surprised and relieved when three of his group replied saying that something similar happens to them. This made it easier for Jess to talk with his friends about this when he next saw them.

Luke had to do a talk to his class for his exams. He felt really nervous. He worried that he would go red and that everyone would notice and laugh and say he was stupid.

Luke felt embarrassed talking about this but decided to tell his teacher, Mr Pye. Luke thought that if Mr Pye understood his worry, he would let him off the talk. Mr Pye listened to Luke and asked him to present his talk to him on his own. Mr Pye thought it was really good and didn't notice Luke going red at all. He suggested that they do a survey. Luke would present his talk, and Mr Pye would ask the class to write down one thing they noticed about Luke's presentation and to rate how interesting they found his talk.

Luke was very nervous, but with Mr Pye's encouragement gave his talk. The feedback from the survey was really positive. Two people said that Luke looked nervous, but no one said anything about him being red in his face. People said that he was easy to hear, spoke well, knew what he was talking about, and rated his talk as 8/10 for interest. Hearing this helped Luke to discover that although he worried about going red, other people didn't notice this, and they didn't think he was stupid.

Surveys can help to discover new information which can lead you to think in different ways.

Responsibility pies

We often blame ourselves for things that go wrong and overlook some of the many other reasons why things happen.

At these times, it can be helpful to make a **pie chart** which includes all the possible reasons why something might have happened. Each reason is given a slice of pie with the size of the slice depending on how much you think it contributed to what happened.

Jade blamed herself for her mum and dad separating. Jade couldn't stop thinking that if she had behaved better her parents wouldn't have argued and would still be together. The more she thought, the more she blamed herself and the worse she felt.

Jade wrote down as many of the possible reasons for her parent's separation she could think of.

▶ Jade had been difficult and her parents did argue about her behaviour.

▶ They also argued about lots of other things – money, who did what around the house, how much time they each spent with their friends.

▶ Mum and Dad split up last year and were always arguing about who was to blame.

▶ Dad's mum was always interfering and telling mum she was not doing things right which caused lots of arguments.

▶ Dad had recently lost his job and seemed to be angry all the time.

▶ They had lots of bills to pay, and dad wouldn't do anything to sort them out.

Jade put these into her pie chart and divided up the slices to show how much each one was responsible for her parents separating. The final slice, her behaviour, was left to the end after the other slices had been sorted.

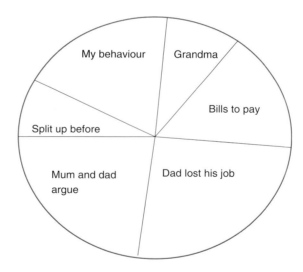

This helped Jade to get things in perspective. Her parents did argue about her behaviour, but there were many other, more important reasons that caused them to separate.

If you are blaming yourself for something, try to get things in perspective with a responsibility pie.

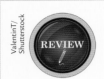

If you find it hard to challenge your thoughts, do an experiment to check out your beliefs and predictions.

Experiments are powerful ways to check out your thoughts and to discover new information.

Surveys and searches can help you check whether there might be different ways of understanding and thinking.

Responsibility pies can help you put things in perspective.

Experiments can help to put some limits around our thoughts and help us discover different way of understanding the things that happen.

Check it out

If you notice strong thoughts that are hard to change try doing an experiment to check out what actually happens.

Step 1: What is the thought to test?

How much do you believe it? (1–100)

Step 2: What experiment could you do to test this thought?

Step 3: What do you think will happen?

Step 4: What happened?

Step 5: What have you found out?

Step 6: Has this changed your belief or prediction?

How much do you believe the thought you tested? (1–100):

Surveys and searches

Surveys and searches can help you check whether there might be different ways of understanding and thinking about things.

My belief or assumption to test:

What survey or Internet search can I do to check this out?

What did I find out in the survey or search?

How does this fit with what I believed or assumed?

Responsibility pie

We often blame ourselves for things that go wrong and overlook the many other reasons why things happen. To keep things in perspective, try making a responsibility pie.

Think about all the possible reasons why something might happen and give each a slice of the pie. The more the responsibility, the larger the slice.

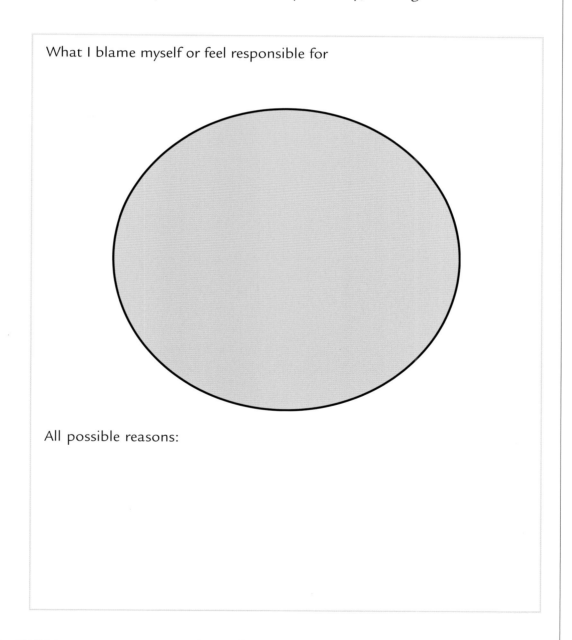

What I blame myself or feel responsible for

All possible reasons:

Face your fears

We often avoid or put off doing things that make us feel anxious. Often, we would really like to do these things, but our worries and anxious feelings take over and stop us.

▶ You may **want** to have more friends, but if you worry about talking with people, you may **avoid** social situations.

▶ You may **want** to go to new places, but if you worry about going somewhere unfamiliar, you may **avoid** going.

▶ You may **want** to join a club, but if you worry about performing in front of others, you may **avoid** going to a sports trial or a musical or an acting audition.

Avoiding things may make you feel better in the short term, but in the long term, it doesn't help.

Avoidance limits what you can do.
You don't have a chance to do the things you would like to do.

You don't learn to cope.
You never learn to beat your worries and to face your fears.

You still feel bad.

Although you may not feel so anxious, if you avoid things, you will still have to cope with other unpleasant feelings. You may feel sad as you spend a lot of time on your own, frustrated that you can't go to new places, or angry that you can't join a club.

Thinking Good, Feeling Better: A Cognitive Behavioural Therapy Workbook for Adolescents and Young Adults, First Edition. Paul Stallard.
© 2019 John Wiley & Sons Ltd. Published 2019 by John Wiley & Sons Ltd.
Companion website: www.wiley.com/go/thinkinggood

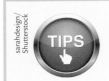

TIPS

Instead of avoiding things that make you feel anxious, you need to reclaim your life. You can do this by taking **small steps** to climb your **fear ladder** to **face your fears**.

Small steps

Facing the things that make you anxious may seem very hard to do. To make it easier, it can be helpful to break your fears in to **small steps**.

What is you fear?

Think about the things you fear, and choose one that you would like to do battle with. It could be the following:

- Social situations

- Spiders, snakes, or animals

- Crowded, high, or enclosed places

- Germs or dirt

What do you avoid?

Think about all the specific situations or things that your fear makes you avoid.

- If you are very anxious in social situations, you might avoid going to parties, talking in class, telephoning a friend, or sitting with people at lunchtime.

- If you are fearful of dogs, you may avoid visiting people with dogs, going into parks, public spaces, or cross the road if you see a dog.

- If you are very anxious in crowds, you might avoid going to town, the cinema, school assemblies, or travelling on buses.

- If you are very anxious about germs or dirt, you might avoid using public toilets, touching door handles, sitting in certain places, or using a shared computer.

What would you like to do?

What would you like to do after you have beaten your fear?

- If you are anxious in social situations, you might want to be able to sit with people at lunchtime.

> If you are fearful of dogs, you might want to be able to visit your friend who has a pet dog.

> If you are anxious in crowds, you might want to be able to go to the cinema.

> If you are worried about germs, you might want to be able to use the toilets at school.

Think about all the things you avoid because of your fear and chose one that you will face and overcome.

Make a fear ladder

Once you have identified what you would like to do (your goal), think about the small steps that will help you to achieve it. You can have as many steps as you like, but make sure that each step pushes you, but feels achievable.

For each step, rate how anxious you would feel if you were in that situation from 1 (not at all anxious) to 100 (worse anxiety possible).

Now create your **fear ladder** by putting the steps in order from the least scary to the scariest.

browndogstudios/ GettyImages

Helen felt very anxious talking with other people and spent a lot of time at school on her own avoiding people. Helen was feeling lonely, and although she felt anxious, she really wanted to have a friend.

Helen wrote down all the situations she was avoiding and rated how anxious they made her feel.

What I avoid	Anxiety 1–100
Travelling to school on the bus	80
Saying hello to someone in my class	40
Sitting next to someone in class	30
Going to the canteen at lunchtime	55
Joining in class discussions	75
Asking a classmate for help with my homework	45
Going into town with others after school	70
Joining in with chat on Facebook	70
Asking someone to go for a coffee	65

Helen thought about what she would like to be able to do after she had beaten her fears. She decided that her first step would be to ask a girl (Sian) to go in to town with her after school. Helen made her fear ladder of small steps that would help her to achieve her goal.

My goal	Go with Sian to town	70
Step 5:	Invite Sian to town after school	65
Step 4:	Go to the canteen for lunch with Sian	55
Step 3:	Ask Sian for some help with her English project	45
Step 2:	Talk with Sian about her English project	45
Step 1:	Say hello to Sian at school	40

Helen didn't feel ready to tackle all the things she was avoiding. Going to school on the bus and joining in with class discussions felt too hard. But by taking a small step and working on her fear ladder, Helen felt she would be able to become more sociable.

Think about the small steps that will help you to face your fear. Arrange them in order of difficulty and create a fear ladder.

Face your fears

The final step is to reclaim your life by facing the first step on your fear ladder. Once you have faced and learned to cope with this, move up the next step on your ladder and keep climbing until you have achieved your goal.

Facing the things that you are avoiding will be hard. You have learned to cope with your anxious feelings by avoiding things. Avoidance brings short-term relief, but in the longer term, you miss out on many of the things you really want to do. By facing your fears, you will discover that

▶ your fears are **not as bad** as you imagine

▶ your **anxiety does come down**

▶ you **can cope** with your anxiety

How do I face my fears?

▶ **Choose a step**. Take the first step on your fear ladder. It is important to start with the step that creates less anxiety so that you can be successful.

- ▶ **Plan**. Write down what you will do, when you will do it, who will help you, and how you will cope. Planning will give you a deadline and will help you feel more in control.

- ▶ **Face you fear**. As you face your fear, **you will feel anxious**. The idea is to discover that your anxiety will come down. To help you notice this rate, your anxiety from 1 to 100 before, a few times during, and after you have faced your fear.

- ▶ **Stay with it**. Even though you feel anxious, it is really important that you **do not leave** the situation or bail out. This is what you have done in the past, and it doesn't help. Wait until your anxiety rating has come down, before you leave. It will come down!

- ▶ **Practice**. Your anxiety won't suddenly disappear after facing your fear once. The more you practice, the less anxious you will become.

- ▶ **Take the next step**. When you feel that you can successfully cope, move on to the next step of your fear ladder.

- ▶ **What have you discovered?** After you have faced your fear, think about what you have discovered. If you stay in the situation, **anxiety will reduce** and you are **able to cope**. Now celebrate what you have achieved and give yourself a treat.

Although you will feel anxious, you can beat you anxiety by facing your fears and learning to cope with your anxious feelings.

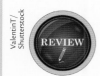

ValentinT/ Shutterstock

By avoiding things, you never learn to cope with your anxiety. Take your anxiety with you, and don't let it stop you doing what you really want to do.

Break you fears in to small steps, and chose one of the things you are avoiding to overcome.

Think about the small steps that will help you to face this fear and create a fear ladder.

Start with the first step on your fear ladder and face your fear. Stay with it until your anxiety has come down.

Move on to the next step and continue up your fear ladder until you have achieved our goal.

Small steps

Think about your fears, and write down all the specific situations or things your fear makes you avoid:

My fear

I avoid

I avoid

I avoid

I avoid

I avoid

I avoid

I avoid

I avoid

I avoid

Fear ladder

Decide which of your small steps, you would like to tackle (your goal) and write it at the top of the ladder.

Think about the steps that will help you reach your goal and rate each from 1 (not at all anxious) to 100 (worse anxiety possible) and put them in order from the least to the most scary.

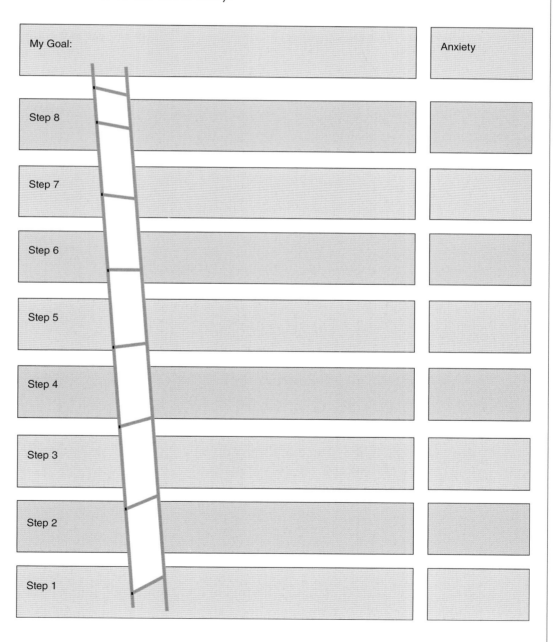

My Goal:	Anxiety
Step 8	
Step 7	
Step 6	
Step 5	
Step 4	
Step 3	
Step 2	
Step 1	

Face your fears

Chose the first (least scary) step from your fear ladder and decide when you will face it. You will feel anxious, but you need to take the anxiety with you rather than letting it stop you from doing things.

You may want to practice each step a few times before moving up your ladder to the next step.

The step I will take

When I will do it?

What happened to my anxiety? (Rate 1–100)

How anxious I felt before I faced my fear:

How anxious I felt whilst I faced my fear:

How anxious I felt after I faced my fear:

What have I discovered?

What step will I take next?

What I will do to celebrate my achievement

Get busy

When you feel down, it can be very hard to motivate yourself. Everything feels too much of an effort. You

▶ **Go out less**.

▶ Spend **less time with people**.

▶ **Stop doing things** that you used to enjoy.

▶ Have **fewer opportunities to enjoy** yourself.

▶ Spend **more time on our own**.

sarahdesign/
Shutterstock

The less you do, the more thinking time you have, the more you think in unhelpful ways, and the worse you feel.

You will become stuck in your **thinking traps** and find yourself:

Rehearsing what has happened and thinking how bad it was

▶ You only think about the bad things that happen (negative glasses).

▶ You make small things bigger than they really are (blowing things up).

▶ You blame yourself for everything that goes wrong (blame me).

Worrying about what will happen and how bad it will be

▶ You expect things to go wrong (fortune teller).

▶ You worry that people will be thinking bad things about you (mind reader).

▶ You worry that you won't be perfect (expect to be perfect).

Thinking Good, Feeling Better: A Cognitive Behavioural Therapy Workbook for Adolescents and Young Adults, First Edition.
Paul Stallard.
© 2019 John Wiley & Sons Ltd. Published 2019 by John Wiley & Sons Ltd.
Companion website: www.wiley.com/go/thinkinggood

Catching, checking, challenging, and changing your thoughts can be helpful, but it may be hard to do if you are feeling particularly down. Your thoughts might seem unstoppable and overwhelming.

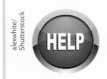

RFvectors/ Shutterstock

Getting busy

Instead of challenging your thoughts, you can help yourself to feel better by changing your behaviour and by **getting busy**. This will help you to do more of the fun things you enjoy and find rewarding.

alexwhite/ Shutterstock

To start with, you may find it hard to motivate yourself. You will probably feel tired and will find many excuses not to do things. You will have to push yourself to get going and the ideas below may make it easier.

Choose activities that are important for you. Think about the things that will make a real difference to how you feel. Choosing these will help you feel more motivated to try.

Take it slowly. You probably haven't done much for a while, so don't be too ambitious. Choose small tasks to make sure that you are successful.

Do it now. Don't wait until you feel like doing it. It doesn't matter how you feel. Set a day and time and do it.

Celebrate success, no matter how small. Be kind and praise yourself.

Acknowledge what you have achieved. Resist the temptation to put yourself down by focusing on the things you still have to do. Think what you would say to your best friend if they had taken the first small steps to reclaiming their life.

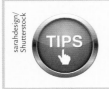

sarahdesign/ Shutterstock

The aim is to get busy, so don't expect to feel better straightaway. It may take a little time before the enjoyment returns.

What you do and how you feel

To help you find out more about what you do and how you feel, try to keep a diary. Chose a couple of days and write down each hour:

▶ **What you were doing**, where you were, who was there?

▶ **How you were feeling**?

▶ **How strong the feeling was?** Rate this from 1 (very weak) to 100 (very strong).

After you have completed the diary, **look for any patterns**:

▶ What were you doing when you were feeling really bad?

▶ Were there times when the feelings were less strong?

▶ What were you doing at the times you felt better?

brown dogstudios/
Getty Images

Jason had been feeling low for several months and really wanted to change how he was feeling. For each hour of the day, he wrote down what he did and how he felt.

Day and time Monday	What were you doing, where, who with	How did you feel	How strong was the feeling?
7 am	In bed, on my own	Sad	85
8 am	Getting ready for college	Sad	85
9 am	Walked to college on my own	Sad	90
10 am	Maths, couldn't understand it	Sad	100
11 am	English, working with Jed and Sara	OK	60
12	PE. Circuit training	OK	50
1 pm	Dinner time with Jed	OK	55
2 pm	Science, experiments in groups with Tom and Seb	OK	55
3 pm	Geography	Sad	60
4 pm	Went to shops with Adil and Tara	OK	55
5 pm	Made an excuse to go home. No one else here when I arrived	Sad	80
6 pm	Tea, ate in my room on my own	Sad	80
7 pm	In bedroom on own watching TV	Sad	85

(*continued*)

(*Continued*)

Day and time Monday	What were you doing, where, who with	How did you feel	How strong was the feeling?
8 pm	In bedroom on own watching TV	Sad	90
9 pm	Online gaming with Jack	OK	50
10 pm	Online gaming with Jack – lost!	OK	60
11 pm	Bed, couldn't sleep, worrying about school	Sad	80
12 pm	Bed, worrying about school	Sad	90

When Jason looked at his diary he found that

▶ it confirmed that he was feeling sad. He hadn't felt happy all day.

▶ his mood changed throughout the day. He felt worse in the morning and evening and better during the afternoon.

▶ he felt better when he was with people doing things (going to the shops, eating dinner, and gaming)

▶ although Jason made excuses to avoid being with his friends, he felt more unhappy (80) at home than when he was with them (55).

Keep a diary to check the link between what you do and how you feel.

Change what and when you do things

Understanding the times you feel particularly bad and the activities that make you feel better or worse can help you **plan to do things differently**.

The diary showed that Jason's mood dropped when he returned to an empty house at the end of the day and was better when he was in PE. Jason liked sport and decided that he would change what he did when he returned home. Instead of staying at home on his own, he would go for a run.

Mornings were difficult for Jason. His mood was low as he walked to school on his own. Although he worried about being with his friends, Jason often felt better when we was with other people. Jason decided to change things around and arranged to meet up with his friend Jed and walk to school with him.

You can't change everything. Jason felt really down in maths, but he couldn't stop going to his maths lesson. Focus on changing the things you can do something about.

Have more fun

When you feel down, you will probably feel tired and have little energy. You stop doing things, even the things you used to enjoy. There is no reason why you wouldn't enjoy these things again, so try to **build them back** into your daily routine.

Make a list of the things:

▶ you used to enjoy but have now **stopped doing**.

▶ that you enjoy but **don't do very often**.

▶ that you haven't done but **would like to do**.

Think carefully about the things that **involve people**. Being with other people provides you with the chance to get busy and to socialise. Think about what you could do with others. It could be

▶ shopping with your sister

▶ going to the cinema with your friend

▶ eating with your family

▶ meeting a friend in a cafe

Give you a **sense of achievement**. Think about the things that give you a sense of pride and accomplishment. It could be anything like

▶ drawing

▶ playing an instrument

▶ fixing your bike

▶ sorting out your clothes

▶ completing a puzzle

Think about the things that **you really enjoy**. This depends on you and could be things like

▶ gaming

▶ cooking

▶ listening to music

▶ reading

▶ watching a DVD

Get active. This could be something energetic like

▶ running

▶ dancing

▶ swimming

▶ a work out

▶ a walk

▶ sorting your bedroom

From your list, decide on one or **two things** you will do this week. These should be things that are important to you, give you a sense of achievement, and are achievable.

Don't try and do too much. The idea is to **be successful** so set yourself small targets. It is better to set a target like playing your guitar once for five minutes rather than practicing for an hour.

At the end of each week, **celebrate what you have achieved** and build on what you have done. For example you could set yourself a target to play your guitar twice per week for five minutes or introduce another goal like phoning a friend.

Find the activities that are important and enjoyable for you and start to build them into your daily routine.

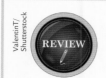

REVIEW

Understand the link between what you do and how you feel.

The less you do the more time you have to worry about what has and will happen.

Get busy and do more of the fun things that you enjoy.

Change what and when you do things. Do things that make you feel better at the times you feel worse.

You can feel better by becoming busier and by doing more activities that lift your mood.

What you do – how you feel

Check out the link between what you do and how you feel. Fill out this diary for a few days and rate your feeling throughout the day.

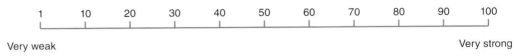

1   10   20   30   40   50   60   70   80   90   100

Very weak   Very strong

Day	What were you doing, where, who with	How did you feel	How strong was the feeling?
7–8 am			
8–9 am			
9–10 am			
10–11 am			
11–12 am			
12–1 pm			
1–2 pm			
2–3 pm			
3–4 pm			
4–5 pm			
5–6 pm			
6–7 pm			
7–8 pm			
8–9 pm			
9–10 pm			
10–11 pm			
11–12 pm			
12–1 am			

Are there any patterns? What are you doing when your unpleasant feelings are strong and when they are weak?

Have more fun

When we feel down we stop doing things, even the things we enjoy. Write down the fun and important things for you.

What I used to like doing but have stopped

What I like, but don't do very often

What I want to do

What is important to you and would help you to start to reclaim your life?

Plan more fun

Choose two or three things you would like to do during your week. Try to get a mix of things that you **enjoy**, are **active**, involve **people**, and which give you a sense of **achievement**.

Plan them in your diary and write down what you actually did.

	What I will do	What I did
Monday		
Tuesday		
Wednesday		
Thursday		
Friday		
Saturday		
Sunday		

CHAPTER NINETEEN

Keeping well

To keep well, you need to make sure that you keep using the ideas and skills that you have found helpful. To make sure that you don't slip back into your old unhelpful ways, it can be useful to make a **keeping well plan**. Think about

- ► **What helped**

- ► **Build them into your life**

- ► **Practice them**

- ► **Expect setbacks**

- ► **Know your warning signs**

- ► **Watch out for difficult times**

- ► **Be kind to yourself**

- ► **Stay positive**

What helped?

There will be some ideas you found helpful and others that just didn't work for you. To make sure you don't forget, write down the important things you discovered and the things that were helpful for you.

Important messages I discovered?

- ► Avoiding things doesn't help you learn to cope.

- ► Thoughts are like waves which come and go.

- ► The less you do, the more time you have to think.

Ideas I found useful?

- ► Breaking challenges into smaller steps.

Thinking Good, Feeling Better: A Cognitive Behavioural Therapy Workbook for Adolescents and Young Adults, First Edition. Paul Stallard.
© 2019 John Wiley & Sons Ltd. Published 2019 by John Wiley & Sons Ltd.
Companion website: www.wiley.com/go/thinkinggood

- Mindful walking.

- Doing something to look after yourself when you feel down.

What helps me relax and feel better?

- Physical activity.

- Speaking to yourself in a kinder way.

- Your soothing toolbox.

What helps me cope with my thoughts?
You may have found mindfulness helpful or preferred challenging your thoughts. What worked for you?

- Watching out for my negative glasses thinking trap.

- Treating myself like I would treat a friend.

- Looking for the positive things that happen.

Write down the important skills and message that you have discovered so that you can remind yourself about what worked for you.

Build them into your life

To encourage you to use your skills, look for ways in which you can build them into your life. The more they become part of your daily or weekly routine, the more you will be reminded to use them.

Build your skills into your daily routine.
Try to link using your skills with the tasks or events that happen each day.

- As you get dressed in the morning, can you scan for any unhelpful thoughts and challenge any thinking errors?

- As you brush your teeth, can you practice speaking kindly to yourself?

- At lunchtime, can you practice being mindful?

- Before you eat in the evening, can you find one positive thing that has happened today?

- As part of your night-time routine, can you use your relaxation skills?

Remind yourself to use them.

You can write messages or, if you don't want people to know, use objects as a way to remind you to do things.

▶ Write a message on a card in your clothes drawer saying, 'catch, check, challenge, change'.

▶ Tape a message on your toothbrush reminding you to be 'kind'.

▶ Put a message in your lunch box saying 'be mindful'.

▶ Set a reminder on your phone before you eat in the evening to 'find one positive'.

▶ Leave an object on your pillow each morning to remind you to 'relax'.

 TIPS

Building your helpful skills into your life will prompt you to use them.

Practice

When things are going well you may feel less of a need to practice your skills. It is probably your new skills that have helped you to feel better. If you don't practice using them, you may slip back into your old unhelpful ways.

To keep well you need to practice.

The more you practice, the more your skills will become part of everyday life and the better equipped you will be to deal with future challenges.

Review how you are doing

▶ Make a time each week to check what skills you have been practising.

▶ Praise yourself for what you have done.

▶ Think about what might have stopped you from using your skills.

▶ Plan how you can overcome these barriers.

▶ Decide if there are some skills that might be particularly useful to focus on in the coming week.

Review how you are doing each week to make sure that you are practising the skills you found helpful.

Expect setbacks

Life is full of surprises, but one thing is for sure – **unexpected problems and challenges will keep coming**. Your new skills won't stop them from happening, so expect to be challenged.

When you are faced with challenges, you might find yourself briefly slipping back into your old unhelpful ways. Don't worry. This is often a short-term slip and does not mean that your old habits have taken over again. Notice what is happening and use your helpful habits.

Short-term setbacks are normal, so don't worry. If this happens, make an extra effort to use your new skills.

Know your warning signs

To make sure that you don't slip back and become trapped in your old unhelpful ways, make a list of the warning signs you need to look out for. These might be

Your old unhelpful ways of thinking.

▶ Arguing with your thoughts may be a warning sign that you are struggling to be mindful.

▶ Focusing on the negative things that happen may be a warning sign that you are becoming caught in your old thinking traps.

Body signals associated with unpleasant feelings.

▶ Racing heart and feeling hot may be warning signs that your anxiety is increasing.

▶ Being tearful and finding it hard to sleep may be warning signs that your mood is dropping.

Ways of behaving that might make things worse.

▶ Spending more time in your room on your own may be a warning sign that your mood is dropping.

▶ Beginning to avoid things may be a warning sign that your anxiety is increasing.

The better you are at noticing your warning signs, the sooner you can do something to change this.

 Watch out for difficult times

There will be times when you have to deal with situations or events that you will find difficult to cope with.

▶ If you have high standards, you might expect to have more anxious thoughts and feelings whilst preparing for exams.

▶ If you find social situations difficult, you might expect to feel more anxious when you have to go to a large social gathering or to talk with people you don't know very well.

▶ If you don't like change, you may find it difficult when you have to go somewhere new.

▶ If you have a lot of time on your own, you might expect your mood to drop as you spend more time listening to your negative and unhelpful thoughts.

Being better at **spotting difficult situations** gives you a chance to **plan** how you will deal with them and to **practice the skills** that will help **you cope.**

▶ Whilst preparing for exams make a revision timetable and practice your relaxation skills before you start revising.

▶ If meeting a group of new people, practice what you might talk about and focus on what they are saying rather than how you are coming across.

▶ If you are going somewhere new try to think of this positively, and remember how you coped with previous changes.

▶ If you have more thinking time, try to build in time to practice your mindfulness.

Watch out for challenging situations, and plan how you will cope and the skills you need to practice.

Be kind to yourself

It is very easy during a setback to slip back into your old ways and to beat yourself up. You may

 start to **criticise** or call yourself names

 blame yourself for letting this happen

 focus on your **faults**

Remember, things **will go wrong**, you are not perfect, you will make mistakes, and unkind things happen.

Accept what happens and don't blame yourself.

Accept what happens, be patient, and treat yourself kindly.

Stay positive

Setbacks are a normal part of life. Many are short-term problems which can be quickly dealt with by using your skills. Because you had a setback does not mean that your problems are back or that your skills no longer work.

If you are having a setback, it is the time to practice using your new skills even more. They have been useful before, so there is no reason why they can't help again.

 Stay positive and remind yourself that

 You can beat this – you were able to beat this last time you can do it again.

 Remember your strengths – focus on the skills and strengths you have that will help.

- **Focus on what you achieve** – notice what you have been able to achieve no matter how small.

- **Reward yourself** – praise yourself for continuing to change.

Focusing on your strengths and what you achieve will help you to keep fighting your problems.

When do I need to get help?

There may be times when you end up trapped in your old unhelpful ways. You might notice that your old habits have returned and no matter what you try you just can't change them.

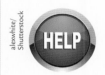

alexwhite/
Shutterstock

When you feel stuck, it is helpful to talk with someone else about how you are feeling. Don't put it off. The quicker you do something, the sooner you will start to feel better.

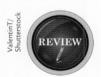

ValentinT/
Shutterstock

To keep yourself well, try to remember what you have found helpful.

Find ways to practice your new skills and to build them into your life.

Watch out for your warning signs and prepare for difficult situations.

Expect setbacks and remain positive. Your skills will help you to stay well.

Keeping well

Think about what you have found helpful and write them down below

Important messages to remember:

Ideas I found helpful:

What helps me relax?

What helps me cope with my thoughts?

This will remind you what you need to practice to keep well.

My warning signs

Make a list of the warning signs you need to look out for that might tell you that you are slipping back into your old unhelpful ways.

My unhelpful ways of thinking:

My body signals and how I feel:

Changes in my behaviour and what I do:

**The better you are at noticing your warning signs, the quicker
you can do something to stop things from getting worse.**

Difficult situations

Think about the situations and events that you will have to deal and plan how you will cope with them.

> What difficult events or situations will I face in the next six months?

> What is my coping plan?

> What skills do I need to practice to help me be successful?

Identifying and planning how you will cope with future challenges will help you to be successful.

References

Bandura, A. (1977). *Social Learning Theory*. Englewood Cliffs, NJ: Prentice-Hall.

Barrett, P.M. (2005a). FRIENDS for Life: Group Leaders' Manual for Children. Barrett Research Resources Pty Ltd.

Barrett, P.M. (2005b). FRIENDS for Life: Group Leader's Manual for Youth. Australian Academic Press Brisbane.

Beck, A.T. (1963). Thinking and depression: I. Idiosyncratic content and cognitive distortions. *Archives of General Psychiatry* 9(4): 324.

Beck, A.T. (1964). Thinking and depression: II. Theory and therapy. *Archives of General Psychiatry* 10(6): 561–571.

Beck, A.T. (1976). *Cognitive Therapy and the Emotional Disorders*. New York: International Universities Press.

Beck, A.T. (2005). The current state of cognitive therapy: a 40-year retrospective. *Archives of General Psychiatry* 62 (9): 953.

Beck, A.T. and Dozois, D.J.A. (2011). Cognitive therapy: current status and future directions. *Annual Review of Medicine* 62: 397–409.

Beck, A.T., Rush, A.J., Shaw, B.F., and Emery, G. (1979). *Cognitive Therapy of Depression*. New York: Guilford Press.

Belsher, G. and Wilkes, T.C.R. (1993). Cognitive-behavioral therapy for depressed children and adolescents, 10–18 years. *Child and Adolescent Mental Health* 3(3): 191–204.

Boydell, K.M., Hodgins, M., Pignatiello, A. et al. (2014). Using technology to deliver mental health services to children and youth: a scoping review. *Journal of the Canadian Academy of Child and Adolescent Psychiatry* 23(2): 87–99.

Burns, D.D. (1980). *Feeling Good*. New York: New American Library.

Cary, C.E. and McMillen, J.C. (2012). The data behind the dissemination: a systematic review of trauma-focused cognitive behavioral therapy for use with children and youth. *Children and Youth Services Review* 34(4): 748–757.

Chiu, A.W., McLeod, B.D., Har, K., and Wood, J.J. (2009). Child-therapist alliance and clinical outcomes in cognitive-behavioural therapy for child anxiety disorders. *Journal of Child Psychology and Psychiatry* 50(6): 751–758.

Chorpita, B.F., Daleiden, E.L., Ebesutani, C. et al. (2011). Evidence-based treatments for children and adolescents: an updated review of indicators of efficacy and effectiveness. *Clinical Psychology: Science and Practice* 18(2): 154–172.

Chu, B.C. and Kendall, P.C. (2009). Therapist responsiveness to child engagement: flexibility within manual-based CBT for anxious youth. *Journal of Clinical Psychology* 65(7): 736–754.

Creed, T.A. and Kendall, P.C. (2005). Therapist alliance-building behavior within a cognitive-behavioral treatment for anxiety in youth. *Journal of Consulting and Clinical Psychology* 73(3): 498.

Dodge, K.A. (1985). Attributional bias in aggressive children. In: *Advances in Cognitive-Behavioural Research and Therapy*, vol. 4 (ed. P.C. Kendall). New York: Academic Press.

Ellis, A. (1962). *Reason and Emotion in Psychotherapy*. New York: Lyle-Stewart.

Fisher, E., Heathcote, L., Palermo, T.M. et al. (2014). Systematic review and meta-analysis of psychological therapies for children with chronic pain. *Journal of Pediatric Psychology* 39(8): 763–782.

Fonagy, P., Cottrell, D., Phillips, J. et al. (2014). *What Works for Whom?: A Critical Review of Treatments for Children and Adolescents*. London: Guilford Publications.

Franklin, M.E., Kratz, H.E., Freeman, J.B. et al. (2015). Cognitive-behavioral therapy for pediatric obsessive-compulsive disorder: empirical review and clinical recommendations. *Psychiatry Research* 227(1): 78–92.

Friedberg, R.D. and McClure, J.M. (2015). *Clinical Practice of Cognitive Therapy with Children and Adolescents: The Nuts and Bolts*. New York: Guilford Publications.

Garber, J. and Weersing, V.R. (2010). Comorbidity of anxiety and depression in youth: implications for treatment and prevention. *Clinical Psychology: Science and Practice* 17(4): 293–306.

Thinking Good, Feeling Better: A Cognitive Behavioural Therapy Workbook for Adolescents and Young Adults, First Edition.
Paul Stallard.
© 2019 John Wiley & Sons Ltd. Published 2019 by John Wiley & Sons Ltd.
Companion website: www.wiley.com/go/thinkinggood

Gilbert, P. (2007). *Psychotherapy and Counselling for Depression*, 3e. SAGE.

Gilbert, P. (2014). The origins and nature of compassion focused therapy. *British Journal of Clinical Psychology* 53(1): 6–41.

Gillies, D., Taylor, F., Gray, C. et al. (2013). Psychological therapies for the treatment of post-traumatic stress disorder in children and adolescents (review). *Evidence-Based Child Health: A Cochrane Review Journal* 8(3): 1004–1116.

Graham, P. (2005). Jack Tizard lecture: cognitive behavior therapies for children: passing fashion or here to stay? *Child and Adolescent Mental Health* 10(2): 57–62.

Hayes, S.C. (2004). Acceptance and commitment therapy, relational frame theory, and the third wave of behavioral and cognitive therapies. *Behavior Therapy* 35(4): 639–665.

Hayes, S.C., Luoma, J.B., Bond, F.W. et al. (2006). Acceptance and commitment therapy: model, processes and outcomes. *Behaviour Research and Therapy* 44(1): 1–25.

Hayes, S.C., Strosahl, K.D., and Wilson, K.G. (1999). *Acceptance and Commitment Therapy*. New York: Guilford Press.

Hofmann, S.G., Sawyer, A.T., and Fang, A. (2010). The empirical status of the "new wave" of cognitive behavioral therapy. *Psychiatric Clinics of North America* 33(3): 701–710.

Holmbeck, G.N., O'Mahar, K., Abad, M. et al. (2006). Cognitive-behavior therapy with adolescents: guides from developmental psychology. In: *Child and Adolescent Therapy: Cognitive-Behavioral Procedures* (ed. P.C. Kendall), 419–464. New York: Guilford Press.

James, A.C., James, G., Cowdrey, F.A. et al. (2013). Cognitive behavioural therapy for anxiety disorders in children and adolescents. *Cochrane Database Systematic Reviews* (6).

Kaplan, C.A., Thompson, A.E., and Searson, S.M. (1995). Cognitive behaviour therapy in children and adolescents. *Archives of Disease in Childhood* 73(5): 472.

Karver, M.S., Handelsman, J.B., Fields, S., and Bickman, L. (2006). Meta-analysis of therapeutic relationship variables in youth and family therapy: the evidence for different relationship variables in the child and adolescent outcome treatment literature. *Clinical Psychology Review* 26: 50–65.

Kendall, P.C. (1994). Treating anxiety disorders in children: results of a randomized clinical trial. *Journal of Consulting and Clinical Psychology* 62: 100–110.

Kendall, P.C. and Hollon, S.D. (eds.) (1979). *Cognitive-Behavioural Interventions: Theory, Research and Procedures*. New York: Academic Press.

Kendall, P.C. and Panichelli-Mindel, S.M. (1995). Cognitive-behavioral treatments. *Journal of Abnormal Child Psychology* 23(1): 107–124.

Kendall, P.C., Stark, K.D., and Adam, T. (1990). Cognitive deficit or cognitive distortion in childhood depression. *Journal of Abnormal Child Psychology* 18(3): 255–270.

Koerner, K. (2012). *Doing Dialectical Behavior Therapy: A Practical Guide*. Guilford Press.

Leitenberg, H., Yost, L.W., and Carroll-Wilson, M. (1986). Negative cognitive errors in children: questionnaire development, normative data, and comparisons between children with and without self-reported symptoms of depression, low self-esteem, and evaluation anxiety. *Journal of Consulting and Clinical Psychology* 54 (4): 528.

Lewinsohn, P.M., Clarke, G.N., Hops, H., and Andrews, J. (1990). Cognitive behavioural treatment for depressed adolescents. *Behavior Therapy* 21: 385–401.

Linehan, M. (1993). *Cognitive-Behavioral Treatment of Borderline Personality Disorder*. Guilford Press.

Lochman, J.E., White, K.J., and Wayland, K.K. (1991). Cognitive-behavioural assessment and treatment with aggressive children. In: *Child and Adolescent Therapy: Cognitive-Behavioural Procedures* (ed. P.C. Kendall). New York: Guilford Press.

McLeod, B.D. (2011). Relation of the alliance with outcomes in youth psychotherapy: a meta-analysis. *Clinical Psychology Review* 31: 603–616.

McLeod, B.D. and Weisz, J.R. (2005). The therapy process observational coding system-alliance scale: measure characteristics and prediction of outcome in usual clinical practice. *Journal of Consulting and Clinical Psychology* 73: 323–333.

Meichenbaum, D.H. (1975). Self-instructional methods. In: *Helping People Change: A Textbook of Methods* (eds. F.H. Kanfer and A.P. Goldstein). New York: Pergamon.

Miller, W.R. and Rollnick, S. (1991). *Motivational Interviewing: Preparing People to Change Addictive Behaviour*. New York: Guilford Press.

Muris, P. and Field, A.P. (2008). Distorted cognition and pathological anxiety in children and adolescents. *Cognition and Emotion* 22(3): 395–421.

Palermo, T.M., Eccleston, C., Lewandowski, A.S. et al. (2010). Randomized controlled trials of psychological therapies for management of chronic pain in children and adolescents: an updated meta-analytic review. *Pain* 148(3): 387–397.

Pavlov, I. (1927). *Conditioning Reflexes*. Oxford: Oxford University Press.

Perry, D.G., Perry, L.C., and Rasmussen, P. (1986). Cognitive social learning mediators of aggression. *Child Development* 57(3): 700–711.

Rehm, L.P. and Carter, A.S. (1990). Cognitive components of depression. In: *Handbook of Developmental Psychopathology*, 341–351. Springer.

Reynolds, S., Wilson, C., Austin, J., and Hooper, L. (2012). Effects of psychotherapy for anxiety in children and adolescents: a meta-analytic review. *Clinical Psychology Review* 32(4): 251–262.

Rijkeboer, M.M. and de Boo, G.M. (2010). Early maladaptive schemas in children: development and validation of the schema inventory for children. *Journal of Behavior Therapy and Experimental Psychiatry* 41(2): 102–109.

Russell, R., Shirk, S., and Jungbluth, N. (2008). First-session pathways to the working alliance in cognitive–behavioral therapy for adolescent depression. *Psychotherapy Research* 18(1): 15–27.

Sauter, F.M., Heyne, D., and Westenberg, P.M. (2009). Cognitive behavior therapy for anxious adolescents: developmental influences on treatment design and delivery. *Clinical Child and Family Psychology Review* 12(4): 310–335.

Schmidt, N.B., Joiner, T.E., Young, J.E., and Telch, M.J. (1995). The schema questionnaire: investigation of psychometric properties and the hierarchical structure of a measure of maladaptive schemas. *Cognitive Therapy and Research* 19(3): 295–321.

Schniering, C.A. and Rapee, R.M. (2004). The structure of negative self-statements in children and adolescents: a confirmatory factor-analytic approach. *Journal of Abnormal Child Psychology* 32(1): 95–109.

Segal, Z.V., Williams, J.M.G., and Teasdale, J.D. (2002). *Mindfulness and the Prevention of Depression: A Guide to the Theory and Practice of Mindfulness-Based Cognitive Therapy*. New York: Guilford Press.

Shafran, R., Fonagy, P., Pugh, K., and Myles, P. (2014). Transformation of mental health services for children and young people in England. In: *Dissemination and Implementation of Evidence-Based Practices in Child and Adolescent Mental Health* (eds. R.S. Beidas and P.C. Kendall), 158. New York: Oxford University Press.

de Shazer, S. (1985). *Keys to Solutions in Brief Therapy*. New York: W.W. Norton.

Shirk, S.R. and Karver, M. (2003). Prediction of treatment outcome form relationship variables in child and adolescent therapy: a meta-analytic review. *Journal of Consulting and Clinical Psychology* 71: 452–464.

Skinner, B.F. (1974). *About Behaviorism*. London: Cape.

Stallard, P. (2003). *Think Good-Feel Good: A Cognitive Behaviour Therapy Workbook for Children and Young People*. Chichester: Wiley.

Stallard, P. (2005). *A Clinician's Guide to Think Good-Feel Good: Using CBT with Children and Young People*. Chichester: Wiley.

Stallard, P. (2007). Early maladaptive schemas in children: stability and differences between a community and a clinic referred sample. *Clinical Psychology & Psychotherapy* 14(1): 10–18.

Stallard, P. (2009). Cognitive behaviour therapy with children and young people. In: *Clinical Psychology in Practice* (eds. H. Beinart, P. Kennedy and S. Llewelyn), 117–126. Oxford: BPS Blackwell.

Stallard, P. (2013). Adapting cognitive behaviour therapy for children and adolescent. In: *Cognitive Behaviour Therapy for Children and Families*, 3e (eds. P. Graham and S. Reynolds). Cambridge: Cambridge University Press.

Stallard, P. and Rayner, H. (2005). The development and preliminary evaluation of a schema questionnaire for children (SQC). *Behavioural and Cognitive Psychotherapy* 33(2): 217–224.

Thapar, A., Collishaw, S., Pine, D.S., and Thapar, A.K. (2012). Depression in adolescence. *The Lancet* 379(9820): 1056–1067.

Turk, J. (1998). Children with learning difficulties and their parents. In: *Cognitive Behaviour Therapy for Children and Families* (ed. P. Graham). Cambridge: Cambridge University Press.

Whitaker, S. (2001). Anger control for people with learning disabilities: a critical review. *Behavioural and Cognitive Psychotherapy* 29(03): 277–293.

Wolpe, J. (1958). *Psychotherapy by Reciprocal Inhibition*. Stanford, CA: Stanford University Press.

Young, J.E. (1994). *Cognitive Therapy for Personality Disorders: A Schema-Focused Approach* (rev. ed.). Professional Resource Press/Professional Resource Exchange.

Zhou, X., Hetrick, S.E., Cuijpers, P. et al. (2015). Comparative efficacy and acceptability of psychotherapies for depression in children and adolescents: a systematic review and network meta-analysis. *World Psychiatry* 14(2): 207–222.

Index

Thinking Good, Feeling Better: A Cognitive Behavioural Therapy Workbook for Adolescents and Young Adults, First Edition.
Paul Stallard.
© 2019 John Wiley & Sons Ltd. Published 2019 by John Wiley & Sons Ltd.
Companion website: www.wiley.com/go/thinkinggood